The Truth About TMJ

How To Help Yourself

by

Jennifer Hutchinson

and

Cynthia and Bill Still

1994, Reinhardt & Still Publishers
Winchester, VA 22602, U.S.A.

Copyright 1994 by Jennifer Hutchinson & Cynthia and Bill Still
Library of Congress Catalog Card Number: 94-92040
ISBN 0-9640485-0-7

First printing: February 21, 1994 3,000

Medical Illustrations by Daniel F. Burner III & Daniel F. Burner IV

The Burner Institution, Woodstock, VA

Reinhardt & Still Publishers
Winchester, VA 22602

Printed in the U.S.A.

Table of Contents

Acknowledgements

The most important people in my life deserve far more than my thanks and appreciation for their part in this tremendous undertaking ...

- My wonderful husband, who gave me all of his love, understanding, and patience as I relived so many painful memories.
- My two beautiful daughters, who sacrificed precious time with me and allowed me to neglect them just a little.
- My husband and children together, for putting up with my many moods and just being there for me.
- My mother and grandmother, for giving me advice and helping me put the pieces together to tell my story.

A special thanks to Betsy Burnam for her help in compiling important information for TMJ implant victims.

I owe a huge debt of gratitude to Melanie, my dear friend. Without her, my nightmare would have been far worse.

I know every TMJ sufferer in this country joins me in thanking:

- The late Congressman Ted Weiss, Chairman of the House Subcommittee on Human Resources & Intergovernmental Relations, for taking on the investigation of TMJ implants and helping legitimize TMJ disorders. And

Congressman Edolphus Towns, who has expressed a commitment to continue following up what Congressman Weiss started.

- Writer Barbara Deane, for her perseverance and belief that the TMJ implant story had to be told.
- Terrie Cowley, President of The TMJ Association, who has done more for TMJ sufferers than anyone in this country. This book would not have been possible without her invaluable contribution and unrelenting efforts to help others.

And last, but certainly not least, I would personally like to thank every single one of you who has called or written to The TMJ Association, both sufferers and their loved ones. In sharing your stories with us, you have become an important part of the fight to improve the quality of life of TMJ sufferers across the country.

Dedication

To all TMJ victims: It is my hope that you will find relief from your pain and, through knowledge of the truth and the understanding of people who have been there, you will gain the strength to survive and go on. You are not alone. We're all in this together.

Introduction

by Dr. Henry Wall, DDS,
Former Clinical Professor of Oral and Maxillofacial Surgery,
Emory University Medical School, Atlanta

Jennifer Hutchinson, in concert with Cynthia and Bill Still, have produced a remarkable book, filled with invaluable information and safe, practical self-help tips for the millions of sufferers of TMJ disorder.

The Truth About TMJ: How To Help Yourself has been written by a TMJ sufferer who refused to give up after years of pain and the loss of jaw function. Mrs. Hutchinson's research of the subject has been so thorough that she can now be considered a true expert in the field of TMJ disorders. The common sense advice the book provides can be helpful to both sufferers and family members of patients afflicted with this malady. The book should be read by all who are contemplating TMJ therapy, especially anyone considering any form of surgery for the correction of a TMJ problem.

This indispensable book gives advice on inexpensive remedies, how to deal with chronic pain, and how to find support groups. It provides safe and effective methods of pain relief, explains how to select a doctor and suggests what questions to ask. It also deals with the complex problems related to insurance coverage for TMJ sufferers. It is a compendium of symptoms and methods of treatment which belongs in the library of not only TMJ sufferers, but every professional practitioner as well.

My congratulations go to Jennifer Hutchinson and the Stills for a job well done. My only regret is that the book could not have been written and widely circulated decades ago. Tens of thousands of TMJ patients might have been spared untold pain and suffering.

Preface

by Marvin J. Schissel, D.D.S., Vice-President, New York Chapter of the National Council Against Health Fraud, a lecturer at State University of New York, School of Dental Medicine at Stony Brook, and author of *Dentistry and Its Victims*, St. Martin's Press, New York, 1980.

Medical quackery, long a major scourge of humanity, is something relatively new in Dentistry. In the past, unethical and poor-quality dentists confined their efforts to teeth. But things have changed. In the past 15 years, more and more dentists have crossed the ethical boundary, and are treating far too many patients for "TMJ" problems with a wide variety of unproven, unorthodox and many times harmful remedies.

Things have gotten so bad that some dentists jokingly refer to the TMJ as "The Money Joint." The "TMJ" scam has been described by the former director of scientific affairs of the American Dental Association, Dr. Enid Neidle, as Dentistry's "hottest" area of unorthodoxy and out-and-out quackery.

"TMJ," a "disease" unheard of until recently, now seems to be reaching epidemic proportions. As many as 1,000,000 new patients every year visit medical professionals for treatment of their "TMJ" problems. And the American Dental Association claims that as many as 30,000,000 Americans suffer from some sort of TMJ problem. Certainly, some small percentage of these folks actually have some problem with their jaw joint(s), and an even smaller percentage actually needs invasive treatment, but few indeed in my experience. A scientifically accurate book on the subject has been long overdue, and Jennifer Hutchinson has performed a much-needed public service with this volume.

"TMJ" properly stands for temporomandibular joint, the neuro-muscular "hinge" connecting the moveable lower jaw to the skull. But "TMJ" has come to be used to describe a confusing and non-specific muddle of conditions and symptoms, all allegedly caused by a malfunction of the TM joint. Since the joint is rarely the cause of these symptoms, many prefer the term "TMD" (temporomandibular dysfunction).

Most TMJ quackery is based on the long-discredited "bad bite" theory: the notion that the TM joint is stressed because the teeth can't come together "properly." This supposedly leads to a wide variety of symptoms ranging from pain to a host of diseases. This "bad bite" theory was proposed by Costen in the early Thirties, but completely discredited a few years later by anatomical studies.

Despite this, some dentists still try to treat "bad bite" by grinding the teeth, building up the teeth with dental restorations, or using an invasive "bite-correcting" plastic appliance. These treatments, easy, popular, and lucrative, are neither safe nor effective for most of the conditions diagnosed as "TMJ."

One of the most popular treatments, the plastic bite-altering appliance presumptuously called the mandibular orthopedic repositioning appliance, or MORA, can function effectively as a placebo, but it also can make symptoms worse, and often causes enough deforming tooth movement to require corrective orthodontic treatment. If a placebo is to be used, it is better to use a non-invasive one.

There are several surgical treatments for TM disorders, but the failure rate is high, often leaving the patient in continual intractable pain. Eminent pain researcher, Dr. Joseph Marbach of Columbia University, believes that surgery for TMD is greatly over-utilized, and should only be considered as a measure of last desperate resort, and only if a condition amenable to surgery has been definitely diagnosed. Jennifer Hutchinson was a victim of inappropriate TMJ surgery.

Most every type of headache, facial pain, general discomfort, and even athletic and sexual difficulty has been diagnosed, usually inappropriately, erroneously or fraudulently, as "TMJ." TMJ quacks abuse X-rays for diagnosis. TM joint X-rays are appropriate only when there has been trauma, or a history of trauma, or progressive joint disease, but should not be taken as a routine screening procedure.

Electronic instruments are gaining popularity for TMJ diagnosis and treatment, but elaborate and impressive-looking though they may be, these devices, including ultrasound and TENS, have not been found to be effective for "TMJ" treatment or diagnosis. And TM joint noises (clicking or grinding sounds) are often used to justify a false diagnosis. All those who worry about whether they have "TMJ" should know that joint sounds in the absence of symptoms do not indicate disease.

A major problem with TMD is that it is imprecisely defined and poorly understood, even by dentists and physicians. Many physicians, particularly ENT (Ear, Nose and Throat) specialists, confronted with patients with facial pain they could not diagnose, have sent them to self-styled "TMJ specialists." Patients should keep in mind that there is no recognized specialty in TMJ! And some of those who claim to be will start the patient on the familiar round of unscientific and not-needed TMJ appliances and treatments.

Dubious TMJ-related claims have been flooding insurance carriers. Claims for fees in five figures are received for simple electronic and appliance treatments which have no scientific basis, and when insurance companies balk at paying for these fraudulent procedures, some "TMJ specialists" are using the courts to force compliance. These abuses decrease insurance capital reserves, and translate into higher insurance premiums and reduced dental coverage for legitimate procedures.

And ironically, with all this, there is overwhelming evidence that the myriad of symptoms usually diagnosed as "TMJ" will almost always respond favorably to simple, inexpensive, and non-invasive treatment. Simple exercises, warm compresses, soft diet, and judiciously-chosen placebos will resolve most complaints. Only in a small percentage of cases will additional treatment be required.

Most cases diagnosed as "TMJ" will even improve with no treatments at all. This explains why TMJ quacks have enough success to be able to attract more patients. Testimonials are the prime tool of the quack, and it is easy to get testimonials from those 90% of patients who will improve no matter what treatment they receive. But it is the other 10% of patients — that 10% who really have a TMJ problem, and who require sophisticated and advanced treatment — whom we should worry about. These folks will be devastated by the quacks.

Jennifer Hutchinson was one of those 10%. Her story is touching and outrage-producing, and could be told by thousands of other victims of TMJ quackery. These victims have suffered staggering costs: financially, physically and emotionally. And the outcome? Chronic, intractable pain — a shameful result that has been the lot of so many uninformed patients who have fallen into the TMJ trap.

Jennifer Hutchinson is a woman who has been through the TMJ mill with the usual disastrous results. But there has been one redeeming result from her ordeal: this book. She invites you to share her experiences and those of other TMJ victims and learn from them. The book contains a wealth of helpful advice for those trying to cope with the results of quack treatment, as well as accurate scientific information to steer you to appropriate treatment and keep you out of the hands of unscrupulous medical professionals. Jennifer Hutchinson is to be congratulated for deriving an inspiring and invaluable book from her ghastly experience.

Chapter 1

What Happened to Me and Why

If anybody had told me nine years ago that temporomandibular joint disorder, popularly known as TMJ, would dramatically affect every aspect of the rest of my life and the lives of my family, 24 hours a day, I would never have believed it.

It all started with a sudden, knife-like, debilitating pain in my neck and shoulder that left me unable to turn my head and barely able to crawl out of bed. A dentist, orthodontist, and oral surgeon convinced me that the problem was with my TMJs, or jaw joints. They also convinced me — after trying one irreversible and unproven treatment after another — that surgery was the only answer. And so it went, on and on, until I had endured six operations that cost more than $70,000. With each surgery, I became worse and with each I always thought, "Just one more surgery." And with each new doctor I hoped for that magical cure that would give me back my life.

But there never was one final surgery. And there certainly has been no magical cure. I don't know what the future holds for me — my doctors don't even know. I do know that the last nine years of my life have been filled with pain, fear, and anger. My family has been financially devastated because of my medical bills and it's not over yet. I'm afraid it never will be.

How did this happen to me? That's a question I have asked myself many, many times. Out of ignorance, a blind trust in my doctors, and a desperate search for relief, I succumbed to one "miracle" treatment after another, with disastrous results. I didn't know nine years ago that doctors who treat TMJ don't agree on anything, or that most treatments have never been proven to be safe or effective. And I didn't question what they did because I thought they knew what was best for me. As a good friend of mine once said, "All doctors are excellent salesmen. They all make sense."

In 1986 when my oral surgeon said I needed an artificial disc in my right jaw joint, I had no qualms about his advice. After all, he was my doctor. I even felt fortunate to have this state-of-the-art implant available to me. How wrong I was. I would never have believed that the implant had not been tested — even in animals. I didn't find this out until six years after it was put in my joint. And by then it was too late.

Now I am being medically monitored to see what damage the implant is doing to my jaw joint as well as my body. And my health has never been worse. My doctors can't guarantee I will get better if I have it removed. They tell me I might get worse. Nobody knows. So I struggle daily with the pros and cons of leaving it in, and wonder what will happen to me if I don't have it taken out. I know that my pain is steadily increasing in the right joint, and the things that used to help me no longer work. I'm only 38 years old. How will I feel five, ten, or twenty years from now? How much worse can it get?

Throughout it all, I relive painful memories every day. I can remember spending most of my time in bed, crying and wondering how I was going to make it through the day. I can remember watching my husband doing more and more around the house — meals, dishes, laundry, bathing and changing the baby — as well as going to the grocery store or bringing in fast food so I wouldn't have to cook. I look back at all the long hours he put in at work just so we could pay the bills. And it still wasn't enough.

Perhaps most vividly, I can see the faces of my two daughters as I kissed them good-bye for "one last surgery." My little one clung to me with tears streaming down her face, and my older daughter tried desperately not to cry for my sake. Once, as I was preparing for surgery, she looked at me with fear in her eyes and asked, "Mommy, you could die, couldn't you?"

Another night as I was tucking her into bed, she kissed me as she always does and, with tears in her eyes and a tremble in her voice, whispered in my ear, "I wish you didn't hurt. I wish you never had to hurt again. I would do anything if I could make your pain go away." And always, I picture my mother and grandmother waiting by the phone for my husband's phone call to tell them I was okay, that I had made it through another operation.

Sometimes at night, in my dreams, I see the operating room — all silver and white, and very sterile. It's very cold, and I'm shivering — partly from the cold, but mostly because I'm so *scared*. The next thing I know, I'm waking up in intensive care. I can hear a voice that sounds like it's very far away telling me to take a deep breath, as I struggle desperately for air. And then I'm throwing up from the anesthesia, and it feels like my jaw will break before, mercifully, I fall back to sleep. When I wake up again, I'm in my hospital room racked with pain, smelling the anesthesia and betadine used on the long incision that has sliced open the side of my face. My husband is hovering over me, stroking my hair and holding the pan as I vomit, and telling me he loves me. Then he's gone and I'm all alone in the dark again. Each time these nightmares end, I wake up sweating and thanking God that it was only a dream and not another surgery.

And then there's the pain. There are times when it is so intense that nothing helps — Tylenol, muscle relaxers, moist heat — nothing. I try to will myself to sleep because when I'm asleep, I can't feel the pain. But the blessed oblivion of sleep rarely comes. And all I can do is lie on the bed and cry and wonder how many more times I can go through this much pain.

I hate what TMJ has done to me. I know I am cranky and short-tempered and hard to live with a lot of the time. I get so sick and tired of telling my children to be quiet, that Mommy is in pain and needs to rest. But for my two children, pain is a way of life. They know fear and worry that children should never have to experience.

Children need to feel their parents are strong and will be there to take care of them. It must be very frightening for them to see Mommy so dependent on other people. I suppose I will never fully understand all the many, many ways my problems have affected my two children, perhaps for life.

My little one was not quite two years old when I had my first surgery. She grew up with Mommy going away for days at a time and seeing me hurt and cry and breathe into a paper bag as I went through drug withdrawal. It breaks my heart to see my youngest daughter try to wait on me. Sometimes she'll run and get a blanket to cover me up or hand me my Tylenol or just try to comfort me in her own way. She hugs me very tight and tells me, "It'll be okay, Mommy."

My husband, Peter, has stood by me through it all. Sometimes I become so wrapped up in my own pain and fear that I forget what it does to him. Six times, he has paced the floor of a hospital waiting room — alone and afraid. Peter says his concern for me affects him every minute of every day. And every day he calls me from work, just to see how I'm feeling. He holds my hand when I am scared or hurting or just discouraged, comforting me and telling me I'll be okay. He's always there when I need hope, sharing my tears, laughter, and fears. Facing the hard times together has made them easier to bear.

I've seen my mother and grandmother — 72 and 88 — age many years as they watched me suffer. They've done everything they could to help me. My mother never leaves the house in the morning without first calling to see if I'm okay. She says she would give anything if she could go through the pain for me. And my grandmother has told me that I am the first thing on her mind when she wakes up and the last thing she thinks about before she falls asleep at night.

If only I had known nine years ago what I know now. This would never have happened to me. If only I had known the truth about TMJ. I'll never forget the day I heard it for the first time. It was in 1988 during a telephone conversation with a TMJ sufferer named Melanie. We talked for over an hour. I remember my shock as she cautioned me that my doctors were ruining me, and that I shouldn't go back to Dr. So-and-So because he was one of the biggest quacks in the country. She said that he was only interested in money. According to Melanie, he actually travels around the country teaching other doctors how to get more money out of their TMJ patients. What's sad is that I was still so impressed by doctors, I actually defended him.

Melanie also told me that I had probably never needed surgery, but since I'd allowed my doctors to operate the first time, I was in for a lifetime of surgery and more surgery and more surgery. I didn't even believe her then. But Melanie turned out to be right — about everything. It was even worse than she told me.

It was a real shock to go back to my doctors armed with the truth and have them lie to me when I began asking questions. My orthodontist even tried to keep my x-rays from me when I asked for them so I could go get another opinion. It was an even bigger shock to realize that I should never have had that first surgery, or the second, or the third....

That's when I began my own search for solutions to my ever-worsening health problems. I ended up seeing eight different doctors over the next few years. And I was given eight different opinions about what to do next. Since they all couldn't possibly be right, I made the decision not to do anything — at least for awhile. Eventually I ended up having two more operations to correct my bite and it appears that the second was successful. Several doctors told me they couldn't imagine anything else that would have to be done. After all, I'd had both joints operated on, and I now had a decent bite.

It wasn't until the spring of 1992 that I found out that the artificial disc my oral surgeon had placed in my right joint was only supposed to be temporary. The package insert from Dow Corning said so. But my surgeon didn't seem to be worried. He said he would be able to tell from my symptoms, if and when, my disc ever needed to come out. He told me that he had put the disc in some of his patients 20 years ago and they were still doing fine.

But the surgical damage had been done. And I gradually realized with growing horror, that the consequences would never be over for me. I had to face the fact that I had been ruined. It was a terrible time. But I eventually struggled through it, and made the decision to take control of my life. I learned to accept what had been done to me and make the best of it by focusing on the positive things in my life — a supportive, loving husband, two wonderful children, and a family that will do anything in the world for me.

There will always be more pain, more surgery, more fear, and probably more heartache and disappointment for me. Sometimes it seems as though I can't face the future. But I know that the support of my family and my determination to help other TMJ sufferers will help me get through whatever lies ahead.

I'm especially encouraged when I look back and realize the tremendous power of the simple truth. I can see how <u>one person</u> gave me the means to take some control over my life. It was then that I knew I had to do something to help other TMJ sufferers. I just kept telling myself that if I could keep one person from going through what I had gone through....

I decided to start a newsletter for TMJ patients to share information and ideas. I knew many patients were not lucky enough to have a supportive family and people who understood what they were going through. I felt that a newsletter, in a small way, just might provide a little bit of support for them. So I founded the TMJ Information and Resource Center and began publishing *The TMJ Report*.

I knew almost instantly that there was a desperate need for such a newsletter because of the heart-wrenching letters I got from people I had never even spoken with before. They were so grateful to know that there were others out there who were going through the same thing, and that they understood.

Soon I was contacted by Terrie Cowley, President and co-founder of The TMJ Association, a national advocacy group in Wisconsin. After communicating for several months, we decided we could best serve the needs of TMJ patients by combining our energies and resources. I dissolved my organization and became Vice President of The TMJ Association.

Right now, I take each day one day at a time. Yes, I am frightened — very frightened — about what lies ahead. But I am determined to keep fighting and somehow survive.

I am outraged that unscrupulous doctors ruined my health and left me with chronic pain. But, I have turned my anger into something positive by trying to help other TMJ sufferers through The TMJ Association. Sometimes all we can offer you is the knowledge that you are not alone or crazy, and that someone is out there, fighting to try to change things. Maybe it is too late for some of us, but there is strength in knowing that together we can make a difference. Through a knowledge of the truth, and the understanding of other sufferers who have been there, we can help one another cope with one of the most debilitating and unnecessary sources of pain and suffering known to man.

Chapter 2

The Controversy

I'm not alone with my TMJ pain. Like countless others, I'm a victim of this agonizing, often debilitating malady that is surrounded by so much controversy. I understand the TMJ sufferer who writes: "I have bad days and worse days. But I have no pain-free days. I've had fifteen surgeries, and each time I kissed my children good-bye, I knew I might never see them again. There have been times when I prayed I wouldn't wake up."

That desperate prayer is echoed by hundreds and thousands and millions of other voices across the country — the voices of people crying out frantically for help. There are so many of us. According to the National Institutes of Health (NIH), an astonishing 30 million Americans — 80-90% of whom are women — are afflicted with the TMJ disorder in the United States alone.

According to a 1993 estimate, between 500,000 and 1,000,000 *new* patients seek medical intervention for their TMJ pain *every year* (Fontenot, 1992). Some have nothing more than an annoying click or an occasional twinge in the jaw and escape the medical merry-go-round relatively unscathed. But for too many others, a trip to the doctor is the beginning of a nightmare that destroys lives and tears families apart, leaving many bankrupt, desperate, and without hope.

Although a large percentage of the population manifests some symptoms of the TMJ disorder, the shocking fact is that nine out of ten people get better with little or no treatment. Every year, a large percentage of these people's lives are needlessly devastated by unnecessary, unproven, and unsafe procedures.

That fact may be unbearably painful to those of you who have endured the agony of TMJ surgery. But many experts now agree that the majority of people with symptoms of the TMJ disorder are really experiencing muscle spasms, known as Myofascial Pain Dysfunction (MPD), rather than an actual internal problem within the joints themselves. Pain in the joints or muscles of the face is usually only temporary and simply goes away with little or no treatment. Even when a TMJ disorder becomes chronic, most patient still don't need aggressive forms of treatment (NIDR, 1993).

Although safe and inexpensive treatments are successful in over 90% of TMJ cases (Tilghman, 1994), many doctors simply ignore them. Instead, doctors often steer their patients toward a variety of expensive and invasive procedures that frequently make the condition worse.

People afflicted with the TMJ disorder typically spend years being shuffled back and forth between doctors, searching for relief. As their pain intensifies, they become desperate enough to try anything. Most of these TMJ sufferers spend tens of thousands of dollars on irreversible treatments frequently not covered by insurance. When these treatments have failed, as they so often do, TMJ patients are told they're crazy or that they need to learn to handle their stress. Or a doctor may simply abandon them, saying there is nothing else he can do.

The reason for this shocking state of affairs is that doctors can't agree on the cause, definition, diagnosis, or treatment of TMJ. As a result, TMJ is frequently mis-diagnosed, or over-diagnosed, and there are no standards of care. That's because so little research has been done to find out why the disorder occurs in the first place, or the safety and effectiveness of available treatments once it does. In fact, only 2% of the National Institute of Dental Research's (NIDR) 1993 budget was directed towards TMJ research, despite the huge number of people afflicted with the condition.

Dr. Enid Neidle, former director of scientific affairs, for the American Dental Association (ADA) calls TMJ "dentistry's hottest area of unorthodoxy and out-and-out quackery" (Berry, 1987). And Dr. Harold Perry, DDS, and former Chairman of Orthodontics at Northwestern University in Chicago, agrees. Now in private practice in Elgin, Illinois, Dr. Perry believes that the majority of people diagnosed as having TMJ disorders are victims of "iatrogenic dentistry," or disease created by the dentist (Perry, 1991). In response to these charges, the ADA admits that existing diagnostic techniques for the TMJ disorder are flawed and that conventional treatments remain unproven (ADA, 1989).

Overdiagnosis and Misdiagnosis

Diagnosing TMJ is a major problem for doctors. The fact is, the majority of doctors, whether physicians or dentists, don't know much about TMJ to begin with. Some doctors diagnose TMJ in every patient who has a pain above the waist. Others actually claim that TMJ dysfunction causes ailments such as impotence, scoliosis, menstrual cramps, and a host of systemic diseases. Joseph Marbach, DDS, at Columbia University's School of Public Health, says, "a person without pain or limited jaw movement does not have TMJ" (Marbach, 1986).

According to John Dodes, DDS, there is a big difference

between a sign and a symptom. "A symptom is something the patient relates to the doctor. A sign is something the doctor makes up. False signs are established and people with perfectly healthy joints are told they have TMJ disorders" (Dodes, Oct. 1991). Dr. Henry Dutson, orthodontist in Annandale, VA says, "If you look hard enough, you can probably find some kind of a TMJ sign in almost anybody" (Dutson, June 1991).

Although doctors have recognized the existence of the TMJ disorder for some 50 years, it would appear that it is becoming a more and more popular diagnosis all the time. Droves of doctors are now jumping on the TMJ bandwagon. Are TMJ problems really more prevalent today? It is far more likely that TMJ is simply the new catch-all diagnosis for facial or jaw pain of unknown origin.

Falling Between the Cracks

The dilemma faced by people with TMJ disorders is clearly expressed by a pain management specialist who says that, of all the pain patients he sees, including those with cancer, TMJ patients are the most tragic of all, "Everybody treats them, but they rarely get better because there is no one medical professional who assumes responsibility for the outcome of their treatment."

TMJ disorder falls between the cracks of medicine. No one medical specialty wants to be responsible for it. Despite the fact that TMJ dysfunction is an orthopedic problem, its treatment is usually left up to dentists. Perhaps this is because the symptoms of TMJ are normally located in the head and face. Orthopedists, who treat every other joint in the human body, barely acknowledge the existence of the jaw joint, which is the most complex joint of all. For some inexplicable reason, orthopedists simply won't touch it.

Consequently, TMJ sufferers are sent from doctor to doctor, draining their money and energy. A person with TMJ typically goes from the dentist to the orthodontist, to the neurologist, to the oral surgeon. And that's just the beginning. For many, the quest for pain relief will require visits to the orthopedist, physical therapist, ENT (ear, nose, and throat) specialist, osteopath, chiropractor, ophthalmologist, or general practitioner, and it goes on and on. When sufferers doesn't get better, or ends up worse, they are referred to the psychologist's or psychiatrist's office to deal with their "imagined" pain or their suicidal tendencies.

TMJ: The Money Joint

⟶ Some dentists limit their practice to, or emphasize, the treatment of TMJ disorders, and call themselves "TMJ specialists." A few even base their claim of being a specialist on attendance at a weekend seminar. To be called a specialist in one of the eight disciplines of dentistry, a dentist must undergo at least two years of advanced training accredited by the ADA Council on Dental Education. TMJ disorders is not one of the eight disciplines; therefore, there are no "TMJ specialists!" (Dodes, April, 1991).

There is undoubtedly a lot of money to be made from treating TMJ disorders. In one advertisement I have seen, doctors are urged to purchase a kit that includes enough material to fabricate 25 splints, for $95 (*The Functional Orthodontist*, 1984). The average cost per splint, therefore, to the doctor, is a mere $3.80. The cost to the patient, on the other hand, can be as much as $2000 for the splint and perhaps as much as $100 for adjustments which may have to be done several times a month. Even diagnostic tests can be very expensive. An MRI scan alone can cost as much as $1,000.

And TMJ patients who end up in the operating room can easily spend tens of thousands, if not hundreds of thousands of dollars, especially those who have had TMJ implant surgeries. I have a Silastic implant and I've undergone six TMJ surgeries at a cost of $70,000-plus.

Add to this the cost of prescription drugs required by many patients just to function from day to day, and it's easy to understand why so many are financially devastated. Doctors who treat TMJ, on the other hand, are making a lot of money from the pain of their patients.

Surgery — Who Needs It?

Despite increasing evidence that TMJ surgery creates more problems than it solves, a number of surgical procedures remain popular. In 1991 alone, there were 45,000 open joint surgeries and 100,000 arthroscopies among TMJ patients. There are approximately 600,000 patients in the U.S. that have had at least one TMJ surgery since 1965 (Fontenot, 1992). Yet most experts agree that only five to ten percent of TMJ sufferers need surgery. Many of these are trauma victims or people with failed TMJ implants who desperately need effective surgical procedures.

According to Joseph Marbach, DDS, "The worst post-surgical cases are far worse than the worst cases in their natural, pre-surgical states" (Marbach, 1992).

Dr. Marbach believes that only a very small percentage of TMJ sufferers actually need, or can benefit from surgery. "TMJ surgery should be employed *only* in cases of tumors or ankylosis (frozen jaw). Both of these conditions are extremely rare; thus, the vast majority of surgical treatments are unnecessary. This is especially true in the face of the availability of safe and effective conservative treatments" (Marbach, 1993). According to Dr. Marbach, of 4,000 patients he's seen, he has referred none for surgery.

Dr. John Dodes, DDS, a general dentist in Woodhaven, New York, and President of the New York State Chapter of the National Council Against Health Fraud agrees. "For one thing, it has never been proven that an internal derangement [of the jaw] causes pain; for another, surgery does not work — it makes you worse" (Dodes, Oct., 1991).

Many surgeons attempt to repair or recontour the bones of the jaw joint. Since the early 1970's, oral surgeons have been using a variety of biomaterials to replace parts of the jaw, or even the entire joint. Most of these artificial implants have never been tested and have not been proven to be safe or effective. Although some of them have been recalled due to serious problems, several remain on the market.

The situation has not been helped by the fact that at least one leading medical journal allowed researchers who favored a surgical approach to TMJ treatment to publish glowing reports, yet denied access to competent oral surgeons with dissenting opinions. Even worse, one of the leading oral surgeons in the world was publishing false reports about the success of TMJ implants while owning stock in the company which manufactured them.

Chapter 3

Anatomy of a Disorder

If you're like many TMJ sufferers, you probably know a lot more about pain and despair than you do about the disorder itself. That's not surprising since there's so much conflicting information being disseminated about TMJ by so-called "experts". How do you know who to trust and believe? The controversy surrounding the definition, diagnosis, and treatment of the TMJ disorder has left millions of you adrift amid a bewildering sea of medical misinformation. Truth may seem like an uncharted island you must find on your own without any map or compass. And there's only one way to do it. You've got to start your quest for relief with an intimate understanding of your own body, beginning with your intricate and amazing jaw joints.

What is TMJ?

Technically, the term "TMJ" refers to the *temporomandibular*, or jaw, joint itself. TMJ *disorder* refers to problems with those joints. To avoid confusion, medical professionals now refer to the disorder as TMD, or temporomandibular disorder, and use "TMJ" to identify the joint or joints alone. Since so few people have any idea what TMD means, however, we opted to stick with the old term, TMJ, throughout this book.

The TMJs are the two tiny joints in front of the ears that attach the lower jaw (mandible) to the skull. They allow you to open your mouth, chew, speak, and swallow. Together, they are considered to be the most complex joint in the body. Not only do the jaw joints rotate as other ball-and-socket joints, they translate (move down and forward) and move from side to side, as well. When intact, they are the only two joints in the human body that work together as a unit.

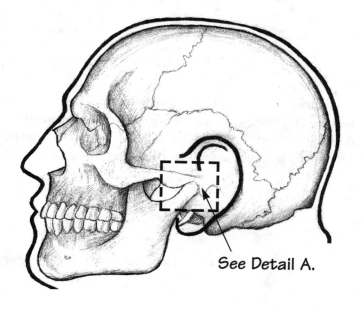

See Detail A.

Illustration by Daniel F. Burner III & Daniel F. Burner IV

The temporomandibular joint contains upper and lower bones. The rounded head of the mandible, called the *condyle*, fits into the hollow of the temporal bone, or the *fossa*. A small, flexible *disc* (sometimes spelled disk), or meniscus, rests on the condyle. The disc separates the bones and prevents them from rubbing against each other, absorbing the shock from chewing, etc.

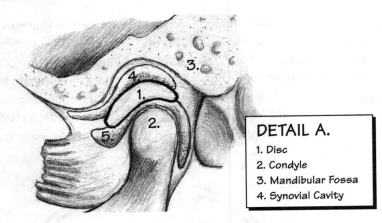

DETAIL A.
1. Disc
2. Condyle
3. Mandibular Fossa
4. Synovial Cavity

Illustration by Daniel F. Burner III & Daniel F. Burner IV

Ligaments help stabilize the joint and keep the bones and disc in their proper positions. Some of the ligaments form a capsule around the entire joint that contains the *synovium*, a lining that produces synovial fluid to lubricate the joint.

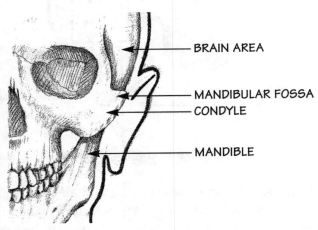

BRAIN AREA

MANDIBULAR FOSSA
CONDYLE

MANDIBLE

Illustration by Daniel F. Burner III & Daniel F. Burner IV

The joint is both stabilized and moved by masticatory (chewing) muscles, such as the *masseter*, *temporalis*, and *pterygoids*. Opening and closing, as well as lateral (side) and protrusive and retrusive (forward and backward) movements are accomplished by these muscles.

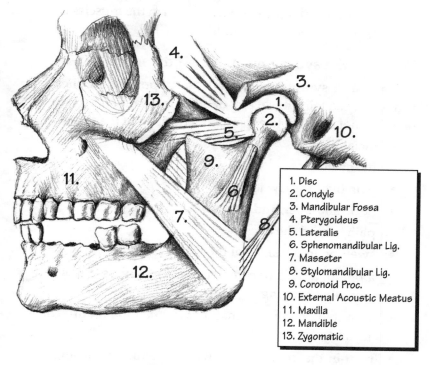

1.	Disc
2.	Condyle
3.	Mandibular Fossa
4.	Pterygoideus
5.	Lateralis
6.	Sphenomandibular Lig.
7.	Masseter
8.	Stylomandibular Lig.
9.	Coronoid Proc.
10.	External Acoustic Meatus
11.	Maxilla
12.	Mandible
13.	Zygomatic

Illustration by Daniel F. Burner III & Daniel F. Burner IV

When the mouth opens, the mandible rotates and slides anteriorly (forward), along with the disc, to a rounded hump on the temporal bone called the *eminence*. When closing, the reverse happens: the mandible and disc slide posteriorly (back).

Although there is so much controversy surrounding TMJ, doctors do concur that the malady is a complex disorder of the jaw joint. Most researchers now agree that TMJ problems fall into one, or a combination of, these three categories:

- *Internal derangement* of the joint (displaced disc and/or condyle, or injury to the condyle)

- *Degenerative joint disease* such as rheumatoid arthritis or osteoarthritis
- *Myofascial pain* (discomfort or pain in the muscles of the jaw, face, neck, and shoulders) (NIDR, 1993).

What are the symptoms of a TMJ disorder?

Signs and symptoms range from popping and clicking sounds in the joint to severe, debilitating pain and dysfunction. It is not unusual to experience one or all of the following:

- facial pain
- headaches
- pain over the jaw joints
- neck, shoulder, and back pain
- pain behind the eyes
- swelling in the sides of the face
- a bite that feels uncomfortable, "off," or as if it is continually changing
- a limited opening or inability to open the mouth comfortably
- pain in the joints or face when opening or closing the mouth, yawning, or chewing
- deviation of the jaw to one side
- the jaw locking open or closed
- sore or worn teeth
- ear pain, ringing, or a feeling of stuffiness or fullness in the ears
- hearing loss
- dizziness or vertigo

The Great Impostor

TMJ has been called "The Great Impostor" because it can

cause seemingly bizarre symptoms that mimic other problems. For example, you may have pain, numbness, or tingling in parts of the body usually thought to be unrelated to the jaw joints and facial muscles.

Much of this confusion can be easily explained by referred pain — or pain that originates in one area of the body but is felt in another. When certain muscles and nerves are injured and/or in spasm, they can cause pain that is experienced at some distance from the original site. In the face, muscle spasms can lead to sinus and tooth pain and pains in the muscles of the neck and upper back. Spasms of muscles in the roof of the mouth and throat can cause changes in hearing, buzzing or ringing sounds, or even dizziness or vertigo.

Although referred pain is often caused by TMJ problems, you run the risk of being misdiagnosed and overtreated when any and every body pain, no matter how remote from the head, is labeled "TMJ." There have actually been cases of patients with Lyme disease, psoriatic arthritis, tumors, abscessed teeth, and even menstrual pains who have undergone extensive, useless, and destructive "TMJ" treatments because doctors mistakenly diagnosed these problems as TMJ. As a general rule, pains in the chest, arms, hands, lower back, and legs should all be checked out by a neurologist before any TMJ treatment is begun.

Clicking and Popping — TMJ Noises

Strange jaw noises sometimes occur when the disc becomes displaced, usually anteriorly (forward). As the mouth opens or closes, the condyle lands, or reduces, on the disc and a click or pop is heard. This condition is known as *anterior disc displacement*, or internal derangement, with reduction. If the disc goes so far forward that the condyle no longer lands on it, the disc gets caught between the condyle and eminence, eventually damaging the disc and possibly the bones as well (osteoarthritis). This is called internal derangement without re-duction, or closed locking, and the clicking becomes a grating sound (crepitus).

Jaw noises are one of the most controversial subjects in the TMJ field. According to several studies, one-third of "normal" joints make noises. It is unknown, however, whether these people will eventually develop a TMJ problem. In some cases, the clicks disappear over a period of time without treatment. Most doctors feel that, if you have no other symptoms, a click or popping sound in the jaw joints is nothing to worry about. Others are anxious to begin treatment and get rid of even the slightest sound. Even though your discs may be displaced, if they are causing no pain or problems with jaw movement, treatment is not necessary (NIDR, 1993).

→ Many doctors use a mandibular repositioning splint which forces the lower jaw into a forward position in an attempt to "recapture" the displaced disc and put it in its proper posi-tion. This type of splint is controversial and can cause irre-versible changes to the bite. [See Chapter 6 for more informa-tion on splints.]

Muscle spasm or joint problems?

The main symptom of muscle spasm (MPD) is tenderness of the chewing muscles (usually bilaterally). If you have MPD you may have good lateral (side-to-side) movement, but a lim-ited ability to open your jaw since the muscles in spasm can cause the disc to be "out of sync." In severe cases, the neck and shoulder muscles may also spasm, causing pain, stiffness, and sometimes numbness and tingling in the arms and hands. You may also hear the infamous clicking and popping jaw sounds so commonly attributed to the TMJ disorder.

If you really are suffering from an internal problem with the jaw joints, rather than muscle spasm, you will usually feel pain over the condyles, combined with restricted lateral jaw movement. Unlike MPD, however, you may have a fairly good ability to open your jaw. In this case, there may be a clicking, popping, or grating sound as your mouth is opened or closed, or while you are chewing. But you should be aware that it is possible to have both MPD and an internal jaw joint problem at the same time.

Chapter 4

What Causes TMJ?

No one knows what causes TMJ. There are only theories. That means that much of what your doctor tells you about your TMJ problem is mere supposition, not fact. The truth is that no one knows for certain what triggers TMJ. *Most* experts agree that there are several different causes of jaw joint disorders. But so little research has been done in this area, that there is still a tremendous amount of controversy.

Dr. Harald Loe, DDS, former director of the National Institute of Dental Research, explains that doctors "have been taught that pain is a *symptom* and the way to relieve a symptom is to remove the cause. If no somatic cause can be found, we may give up and abandon the patient. Or we may hypothesize a cause and treat it, either conservatively or less conservatively. If the treatment fails, we may try something else or tell the patient to learn to live with the pain" (Loe, 1993).

As a TMJ sufferer you know that being told you must "learn to live with the pain" is really no option at all. But I know that far too many of you have probably been told just that. What a doctor really means when he tells you "to live with the pain" is that you're on your own. It means you have to start sorting through the theories about TMJ and decide on your own course of treatment. To that end you should become familiar with the many theories concerning the cause of your TMJ disorder. Some of the most popular of these "educated guesses" are explored below:

Trauma

An injury, such as a heavy blow to the side of the face, or a whiplash, can trigger a TMJ problem.

Disease

The jaw joints are susceptible to the same diseases as other joints in the body, such as osteoarthritis (progressive degeneration of the joint with bony changes, destruction of the disk, and muscle pain), rheumatoid arthritis, gout, and rarely, tumors.

Muscle Spasm

People with TMJ disorders usually suffer varying degrees of pain involving the muscles of the head, neck, and upper back. Some doctors believe that prolonged, recurring, muscle spasm can actually lead to damage within the jaw joint.

The Fibromyalgia Connection

It is believed that many people with TMJ also have a rheumatic illness called fibromyalgia. Unlike arthritis, fibromyalgia does not cause deformities or permanent crippling. Millions of people suffer from the disorder, 80 percent of whom are women between the ages of 20 and 50. The pain of fibromyalgia radiates from the ligaments, tendons, and muscles — the fibrous tissues in the body. As a result, most people with the ailment have extremely tender points throughout their body. Many sufferers hurt all over and are simply too exhausted to hold down a job.

Although the exact cause of fibromyalgia is not known, several factors including viral or bacterial infection, an automobile accident, or the development of another malady such as lupus or rheumatoid arthritis, may trigger fibromyalgia in some people.

In addition to widespread muscle and bone pain, the major symptoms of fibromyalgia include fatigue, disrupted sleep patterns, irritable bowel syndrome (nausea, diarrhea, constipation, abdominal pain and/or gas), TMJ, migraines, and thinking or memory impairment. Certain factors, such as changes in weather, cold environments, hormonal fluctuations, stress, anxiety, and depression can contribute to symptom flare-ups.

Unfortunately, there is no specific test to diagnose fibromyalgia. A diagnosis is based on your medical history, your symptoms, and the exclusion of other disorders. At the present time, there is no cure. And for many people, symptoms simply come and go.

Treatment is aimed at improving sleep, increasing physical fitness (slowly and gradually, with low or non-impact aerobic exercise), and easing pain and fatigue. Physical therapy, especially warm water exercises, the use of hot packs, or other forms of heat, has also been found to be extremely beneficial for some. Relaxation techniques that control stress are important, as well.

Non-prescription, non-steroidal anti-inflammatory drugs (NSAIDS) such as ibuprofen help lessen the discomfort of many sufferers. In addition, your doctor may recommend low doses of antidepressants such as Elavil, or a muscle relaxer such as Flexeril to help you sleep and reduce your pain. But it may take time and perseverance to find out what helps you and what makes you worse.

For more information on fibromyalgia, write to Kristin Thorson, Fibromyalgia Network, 5700 Stockdale Hwy., Suite 100, Bakersfield, CA 93309. [See Chapter 20.]

Genetic/Congenital

Science has yet to determine whether TMJ is inherited. That's because scientists can't agree on what they consider to be an "ideal" jaw structure or position. Everyone's face, jaw, and skull are different. And these differences can be quite normal. The resulting confusion makes diagnosing a TMJ disorder incredibly difficult. The bottom line is that the "experts" simply don't know what anatomical structures or positions of the jaw cause pain or other problems.

Gender

Many epidemiological studies claim that women are more likely to develop TMJ than men, possibly because of differences in their connective tissue, smooth muscle, or cartilage. Other studies find an equal distribution of TMJ symptoms among men and women, yet claim that females outnumber males eight to one in seeking treatment. There is wide speculation as to why this is true. Some feel women utilize the health care system more than men do; others theorize that women have a lower tolerance for pain. But the fact is that most people with TMJ are women between the ages of 18 and 40. This being the case, it would make sense to study the effect of female sex hormones on the development of the jaw joints and TMJ disorders.

Aging

It's a well-known fact that about one-third of people over the age of fifty have some signs of osteoarthritis in their jaw joints. What is not known, however, is whether or not there is a difference in the type of osteoarthritis which is a normal part of the aging process (that affects most joints in the body), and the disease which weakens the temporomandibular joints.

Possible TMJ Triggers

Many practitioners believe there are risk factors for developing TMJ, and that most of them involve situations over which you have some control. If other medical problems have been ruled out, such as allergies, migraines, abscessed teeth, tumors, etc., there is no harm in trying to eliminate some or all of the following factors, which may trigger TMJ symptoms or aggravate an existing problem.

Oral Habits

Some clinicians are convinced that tongue thrusting, mouth breathing, wide yawning, and nail, lip, or cheek biting, can precipitate TMJ problems. They believe that putting the jaw in an abnormal position may weaken and wear down the structures of the joint as well as the muscles. But other researchers feel there is no correlation.

Work Habits/Posture

There are many things people do every day, probably without thinking, that may lead to pain and spasm, either in the muscles of the jaw or those of the head, neck, and shoulders. These include cradling a telephone between your ear and shoulder, typing for long periods of time, talking excessively, carrying a heavy shoulder bag, playing a violin, or anything that causes a forward head position such as hunching forward to read.

Although there is a difference of opinion concerning the part work habits and posture play in the development of TMJ problems, it would make sense to avoid anything that seems to intensify an existing condition or precipitate a pre-existing problem.

Hard Foods/Chewing Gum

People who know they have a TMJ disorder should avoid biting into an ear of corn, an apple, or a triple-decker sandwich, or doing anything that forces the mouth wide open. In addition, it's probably a good idea to stay away from peanuts, Doritos, and pretzels — anything that is hard, crunchy, or chewy (particularly gum).

Dental Work

Certain dental procedures appear to cause symptoms of TMJ in some people. To avoid causing TMJ or exacerbating an existing problem, dentists should not apply too much pressure on the jaw, push the jaw posteriorly (back), or build caps up too thick or fillings too high. Lengthy dental work requiring your mouth to be open very wide for extended periods of time can cause a problem or aggravate a joint predisposed to TMJ.

Many people experience their first symptoms of TMJ after having their wisdom teeth extracted. Although most doctors remove wisdom teeth in their adolescent patients in order to prevent future problems, a recent study shows that most wisdom teeth do not cause trouble and don't need to be pulled out at all (Antczak, 1991).

⇒ Orthodontics

Studies strongly suggest that having orthodontic work done to correct crooked teeth, crowded teeth or a less than "perfect bite" neither causes, nor prevents TMJ. This disputes the widely believed theory that expensive orthodontics will prevent or decrease your chances of developing TMJ.

Intubation

Intubation, or the insertion of a tube into the larynx (voice box) during surgery has been known to cause jaw joint disorders. In this procedure, the patient's mouth must be opened quickly, and very wide, to insert the intubation tube, which may remain in place for a prolonged period of time. If you have TMJ problems and you are contemplating any kind of surgery, you should alert the anesthesiologist so that alternative methods of anesthesia can be considered.

Malocclusion

One of the most common explanations for TMJ is *malocclusion*, or a "bad bite." Proponents of this theory believe that having a bad bite forces your jaw into the wrong position and prevents your teeth from fitting together properly. This supposedly puts extra stress on chewing muscles, causing them to go into spasm, which triggers pain, and still more muscle spasm. The catch is, there is a wide variation in what's considered a good, or normal, occlusion and what constitutes a bad one.

Unfortunately, attempts to correct a bad bite include the use of a number of expensive and irreversible procedures, such as restoring damaged teeth and replacing missing ones, grinding selected teeth, and repositioning the jaw with splints, followed by braces to stabilize the new bite.

Recent research disputes the malocclusion theory, indicating that people with "bad" bites are no more prone to TMJ than people with "good" bites. The fact is, some people with good occlusions get TMJ and some people who have a severe malocclusion never develop TMJ.

Bruxism/Stress

Some doctors tell their patients they have TMJ because they brux (grind) their teeth and that they grind their teeth because they are stressed. But approximately one-fourth of any population — with or without TMJ — grinds their teeth at night (Remba, 1987). Not all people with TMJ grind their teeth, and not all habitual tooth grinders have TMJ. Science has yet to prove whether stress is the *cause* of bruxism and the ensuing pain or merely the *result* of dealing with a chronic pain condition (NIDR, 1993). Another theory of bruxism is that patients with a malocclusion are unconsciously attempting "to find their bite," by realigning their own jaw position.

Perhaps because the overwhelming majority of people seeking treatment for TMJ are women, stress has become one of the most widely-accepted (and most harmful) theories for the cause of TMJ. Women are more likely to be told they have a psychological disorder if they don't respond to treatment, and are blamed for causing and/or maintaining their pain. And with no credible explanation for their suffering, it is little wonder that many of these women begin to feel depressed and alienated from their family, friends, and professional health providers. Some eventually doubt their own sanity.

Can a TMJ disorder be prevented?

Although there is some disagreement about this, most experts believe that taking the best possible care of your teeth might prevent jaw joint disorders that are caused or aggravated by malocclusion (due to missing teeth or excessive dental work, for example). But even if malocclusion has nothing to do with TMJ, taking care of your teeth can certainly do no harm.

According to some professionals, a significant number of children display some sign or symptom of TMJ dysfunction. Parents are led to believe that if their child doesn't have orthodontics, he or she will have a big TMJ problem somewhere down the line. But there is absolutely no proof that early intervention, in the form of expensive orthodontic work, can prevent the development of future TMJ disorders. In fact, some experts feel that jaw problems in young people are related to joint growth, and are just temporary.

Still other practitioners attempt to break thumb-sucking and bruxism habits in children, because they believe they predispose a child to TMJ problems in adulthood. But once again, there is no scientific proof to back up this theory.

The lack of a real explanation for TMJ has set the stage for the current unproven theories about its cause. Many professionals use treatments which are based on their own subjective perceptions of what causes TMJ, resulting in the iatrogenic (doctor-induced) aspect of TMJ. Until scientific studies are conducted to determine the real cause(s) of TMJ disorders, safe and effective treatments will not be developed. If such a cause *can* be found, it might actually be possible to prevent TMJ.

Chapter 5

How is TMJ diagnosed?

With no consensus among doctors or researchers on the cause of TMJ and its symptoms, diagnosing TMJ can be difficult. Presently, there is no standard widely-accepted diagnostic test to correctly identify TMJ disorders. In most cases, a physical exam that includes range of motion tests, listening for sounds in the joints, examining the teeth, and palpation of the jaw joints as well as the muscles of the face, head, neck, and shoulders, should be sufficient for an accurate diagnosis. In addition, it is extremely important for the doctor to ask you questions about pain and other symptoms, past injuries, oral habits, and previous medical and dental treatment.

According to the NIDR, you should only consider expensive diagnostic techniques if you do not improve with conservative treatment or when your doctor strongly suspects you have a condition such as arthritis. Even then, the NIDR advises TMJ sufferers to get another independent opinion, "before undergoing any expensive diagnostic tests" (NIDR, 1993). The most popular types of the imaging techniques used by doctors in the diagnosis of TMJ are described below.

Conventional Radiography (plain x-rays)

Conventional x-rays, such as Panorex, are often the first step in the imaging evaluation of TMJ. These "pictures" show the bony structures of the joint reasonably well, are quick, painless, and acceptably low in radiation. The cost is relatively minimal compared to other studies, usually averaging between $30 and $75.

The main use of conventional x-rays is to rule out obvious pathology such as fracture, arthritis, and developmental deformities.

Conventional Tomography

In Conventional Tomography, a series of x-rays (usually between 4 and 20 per side), are taken. The result is x-ray "slices" of the joint that provide a better view of the bony structures of the joint than plain x-ray films. However, it is more expensive than plain films, and a skilled radiographer is absolutely critical.

Opinions about the value of using tomography varies widely. Some experts feel they are absolutely critical for proper evaluation of a TMJ problem. Others believe they are simply expensive ways to take bad x-rays. It is true that a major drawback of this imaging technique is that soft tissues, including the TMJ disc, cannot be seen on tomograms. But if skillfully done and interpreted properly, tomograms *can* show subtle degenerative or inflammatory changes, and the exact shape of joint structures.

Computed Tomography (CT, or CAT Scan)

CT scanning provides superb detail of the bony structures of the jaw joint using regular x-rays and storing them digitally on a computer. CT offers a way to evaluate the disc without puncturing the joint or using contrast media, and doesn't require a particularly skilled examiner — which are all very desirable features in a diagnostic study. CT scanning is also comfortable for the patient, and the x-ray dose is quite small and limited to the area of interest. It is relatively expensive, however, costing about $300-$400 for both joints, and gives a very limited image of the disc and other soft tissues.

⤳ Arthrography

TMJ arthrography is a diagnostic technique that has been used for many years, and is considered the "gold standard" for the diagnosis of temporomandibular joint disorders. During this procedure, which can be somewhat painful, radiographic contrast dye is injected into the joint. The joint is then imaged using plain x-ray films, tomograms, videotape, or a combination of all three.

If properly performed and interpreted, arthrography can accurately show the anatomy and function of the joint and disc. A wide variety of internal abnormalities such as disc displacements and perforations can be seen.

Risks associated with the procedure include infection from the needle puncture and an allergic reaction to the dye, which are both very rare. A skilled examiner is a must. The cost of arthrography is relatively high ($150 to $250 per side, as a rule).

⤴ Magnetic Resonance Imaging (MRI)

For the last few years MRI has become a popular way to diagnosis TMJ, and is now considered to be the best single way to study the jaw joint. It produces amazingly detailed and accurate images of bone and soft tissues without using x-rays and without injection of contrast dye.

With the exception of a few patients (such as those with pacemakers, for example) essentially anyone can safely have MRI, including children and pregnant women. But MRI can be a lengthy (30-60 minutes or longer) and noisy examination that requires the patient to remain perfectly still until it is over. Some people become claustrophobic and need mild sedation.

Although MRI is costly (average charges can be as high as $1000 or more for a bilateral study), it requires little procedural skill. It is absolutely critical, however, that all studies of the TMJ be done using special equipment (TMJ surface coils) and protocols to allow adequate TMJ examination.

The Trouble with X-rays.

"Imaging can show in exquisite detail the normal and abnormal structures in the joint. It cannot, however, prove that [TMJ] symptoms are related to a particular abnormal anatomy" (Carrera, 1992).

Doctors agree that x-rays do not always provide an accurate means of diagnosis. The trouble, however, lies not with the x-ray images themselves, but with the fallible and subjective opinions of the doctors who interpret them. According to William McCarty, DDS in Montgomery, Alabama, "If a doctor sees what he expects to see on an x-ray, he thinks the x-ray is a good one. However, if the x-ray doesn't show what he was anticipating, then he says it is not a good x-ray" (McCarty, 1988). Dr. Henry Dutson agrees, "If ten doctors or radiologists look at the same set of x-rays, it is quite possible to receive ten completely different reports" (Dutson, 1988).

All this discrepancy can be frightening for the patient. After all, a diagnosis is largely based on what the doctor and/or radiologist sees, or thinks he sees, on an x-ray. If the x-ray is not accurate, how can the diagnosis, and more importantly the treatment, be appropriate?

"High-Tech" Diagnostic Gadgetry

All sorts of elaborate electronic instruments are used to diagnose TMJ disorders, including jaw tracking, surface electromyography, sonography, Doppler ultrasound, thermography, and silent period durations. According to the ADA, none of these "high-tech" diagnostic methods have been proven to accurately diagnose TMJ disorders (ADA, 1989).

One of the most important areas of TMJ research should be developing clear guidelines for diagnosing TMJ disorders. Once scientists agree on what these guidelines should be, it will be far easier for doctors to correctly identify true TMJ problems.

Chapter 6

Questionable Treatments for TMJ

The problem with most treatments for jaw joint disorders is a lack of long-term follow-up studies and good solid scientific research to prove their safety and effectiveness. And although many non-invasive therapies and treatments, such as TENS are considered safe, they also lack scientific validation, and can be enormously expensive.

With far too many treatments for TMJ, it's simply not clear whether people get better as the result of spontaneous remission, a placebo effect, or specific therapies. Another problem is that several treatments are often used simultaneously, so it's virtually impossible to determine which, if any, actually helped. And since most studies are too short, the long-term effects of many treatments are just not known. To make matters worse, normal control groups are usually lacking and the sample sizes are small. The bottom line is that no one actually knows what really works and what doesn't when treating TMJ.

If you get better during treatment, for example, it is difficult — if not impossible — to know whether you improved because of what the doctor did or if you got better in spite of the treatment. Fortunately, the body has an amazing ability to adapt and heal itself in the same way that it can also fight harmful treatments.

Controversial Treatments

According to Donald Tilghman, DDS at the University of Maryland in Baltimore, approximately 80 percent of people who are diagnosed as having TMJ, really have MPD and can be successfully treated with conservative, reversible therapies (Tilghman, 1994). Unfortunately, many patients are ruined by unproven and unnecessary treatments. Some of the more common ones are listed below.

Equilibration

This procedure involves selective grinding of the teeth in an effort to improve the bite. It causes permanent changes in the bite, however, and is not recommended.

Splint Therapy

There are two basic kinds of dental appliances and they differ drastically in their purpose and results. An *occlusal splint* is made of either soft rubber, plastic, or hard acrylic and fits over all, or some, of the top or bottom teeth. The top surface of the splint is flat or smooth, allowing the teeth to find their most comfortable position.

Because using a splint allows the jaws to remain slightly separated, some clinicians believe they enable the jaw muscles to rest, and that clenching, grinding, and inflammation of the jaw joint is reduced. Although many such professionals feel occlusal splints are a safe way of allowing the jaw muscles to relax by redistributing stress, others claim they actually increase the clenching and muscle spasm that can lead to TMJ pain.

The second splint, called a *repositioning* or *mandibular repo-*

sitioning splint, has become controversial because its use can produce permanent, irreversible jaw changes that can be very damaging to your joint. In this type of splint, the jaws are not only separated, but the lower jaw is actually repositioned, usually forward, or anteriorly. The idea is to "recapture" the displaced disc, bringing it back into its proper position. Many doctors expose their patients to unnecessary risk by inappropriately using these splints to get rid of clicking and popping sounds in the jaw joint. But research shows that approximately one-third of the population "clicks and pops" without pain and restricted movement, and no treatment is necessary.

Repositioning splints are based on the unproven assumption that a bad bite and bruxism cause TMJ problems. Dr. Joseph Marbach, former director of the Facial Pain Clinic at the Harvard School of Dental Medicine, and current director of Pain Research at Columbia University School of Public Health, says, "TMJ [disease] responds pretty well to medical management, and that would leave the dentists out. So dentists have developed a whole cult following, based on this notion of bad bite" (Remba, 1987).

These splints are sometimes used to discourage bruxism, which, although unproven, many practitioners claim causes TMJ disorders. But the fact is, twenty-two percent of any population, whether they have TMJ problems or not, grinds their teeth at night. The bruxism theory promotes the use of bite plates (splints) which are worn at night to discourage grinding. According to Dr. Marbach, these bite plates are "basically placebos" (Remba, 1987).

Although splint therapy is very common in the treatment of TMJ disorders, it is controversial and expensive — costing anywhere from $100 to $2,000 — not counting the cost of regular adjustments. "When worn too much, repositioning splints can cause the patient's teeth to move so far out of proper position that orthodontics or facial reconstructive surgery is needed to correct the deformity" (Dodes, April 1991). **Warning**: Any splint that causes or increases your pain should be discontinued.

✝ Orthodontics and Prosthodontics

According to the NIDR, the routine use of braces, crowns, and bridge work to adjust the bite has no scientific basis and is "of little value" in the treatment of TMJ (NIDR, 1993).

Steroid Injections

Some practitioners inject corticosteroids directly into the joint even though long-term use of such drugs can lead to deterioration of the bones, disc, and muscles, and perhaps cause facial paralysis. Like so many treatments for TMJ, steroid injections are extremely controversial.

Surgery

Despite increasing evidence that TMJ surgery creates more problems than it solves, some surgical procedures still remain popular. TMJ surgery is *major* surgery, requiring general anesthesia. It can last several hours, depending on the exact procedure and whether one or both joints are involved.

The basic TMJ surgical procedure is to enter the joint through any one of a variety of incisions, either short or long — from in front of the ear or behind the ear — and make any repairs necessary. The dissection is pretty extensive, and there is a risk that the surgeon will damage one of your facial nerves if he is not extremely careful.

Once inside the joint, if the surgeon finds that the bones of the condyle are rough and irregular, he may decide to try and smooth them down. He may also attempt to repair a worn or perforated disc and secure it in place using a variety of methods. Scar tissue that has formed is often cleaned out in an effort to free the disc and condyle to move more smoothly and increase mobility. The area is then bandaged and you will be sent to the recovery room, usually remaining in the hospital for one to three days.

The extent of immediate post-op pain you will experience depends on the kind of surgery you've received although it can vary quite a bit from one person to another. But you can expect a long and difficult recovery no matter what type of TMJ surgery you undergo.

The trouble with TMJ surgery is that there is a deplorable lack of controlled, scientific experimentation and long-term follow-up proving its efficacy. If you are considering any sort of TMJ surgery, you should be aware that there are a number of serious risks, including *increased* pain, decreased range of jaw motion, jaw bone degeneration, occlusal changes, facial paralysis, and infection.

Since the early 1970s, oral surgeons have been reconstructing TMJs utilizing different biomaterials to replace the disc, or even the entire joint. A variety of materials have been used, including different combinations of metal and plastic. What is so tragic is that most of these artificial implants have *never* been tested and have not been proven to be either safe or effective.

The same is true of autogenous replacements (implants made from ribs and other parts of the patient's own body) which are also commonly used, without proof of their safety or efficacy. As a matter of fact, recent reports of contaminated tissues from tissue banks have prompted the FDA to set standards for such implants, in an attempt to safeguard the public. [For more information on TMJ implants, see Chapter 7.]

When it comes to surgery, one of the few things that most doctors agree on is the importance of post-op physical therapy. Surgery causes swelling, sore muscles, damage to soft tissues, pain, and scarring. Physical therapy is used in an attempt to decrease pain, swelling, and the formation of scar tissue, while increasing range of motion and preventing muscle atrophy.

Such therapy also includes many of the same conservative treatments employed in earlier stages of non-surgically treated TMJ disorders. These include gentle jaw exercises, heat and ice, electrical stimulation, and ultrasound[see Physical Therapy below].

Arthroscopy

Arthroscopy is a surgical technique that was first researched by Japanese oral surgeons in the mid-seventies. Since 1981, however, oral surgeons in the U.S., Australia, Sweden, and Japan, have been utilizing this procedure to exam the jaw joints.

Although arthroscopy *is* a surgical procedure, it is less invasive and expensive than traditional open joint surgery. Two tiny holes, about two to three millimeters in diameter (as opposed to a two-to-three-inch regular surgical incision) are made in front of the ear. An arthroscope, or very small telescope which is linked to a television camera, is inserted in one hole. The second hole is used to remove fluid and debris if necessary.

During the procedure, surgeons can allegedly view problems such as disc dysfunction, tears, or perforations, and soft tissue diseases as well as adhesions (scar tissue). They can also listen to sounds of the jaw in motion to help distinguish between a click caused by a displaced disc, and a grating noise, or crepitus, caused by arthritis. An arthroscope can also be used to wash out debris, cut away scar tissue, or reposition a disc. If there is inflammation, a small amount of steroid solution can be put into the joint.

Proponents of arthroscopy claim it has many advantages. It only takes about an hour, can be done on an outpatient basis, and recovery time is reduced to approximately two weeks. Swelling, scarring, and the chance of bleeding and infection are supposedly reduced. And no sutures are required — just a pressure bandage. Some surgeons are now trying to come up with a way to repair a damaged disc using arthroscopy. Eventually, they hope to be able to insert the arthroscope through the ear canal, eliminating the need for facial incisions all together.

It all sounds so good if you are racked by chronic pain and desperately searching for relief. Unfortunately for TMJ sufferers, arthroscopy is not without risk. One possibility, although rare, is that a piece of an instrument can break off and perforate the joint, then enter the brain. More common risks involve nerve damage or hearing problems. And, as with any surgery, there are always the usual risks associated with general anesthesia.

Orthognathic Surgery

Some doctors try to surgically "rearrange" (reposition and reshape) their patients' jaws during *orthognathic* surgery. By rearranging both parts of the jaw, or just the upper or lower portion, they typically use this procedure in an attempt to correct a severe malocclusion or growth deficiency. Following surgery, most peoples' jaws are wired shut in order to hold them in their new position until they heal. During this time, which usually ranges from one to eight weeks, the patient is kept on a liquid or soft diet. The recuperation period varies, too; some people are back to work in a couple of weeks, while others need several months to really get back on their feet again.

Physical Therapy

Numerous other treatments for TMJ disorders fall into the domain of the physical therapist. Although many of these are considered to be safe, and a number of people with TMJ swear by them, you should also be aware that some TMJ sufferers actually get worse when undergoing physical therapy. In fact, physical therapy has never been scientifically proven to benefit jaw joint disorders.

The primary goals of physical therapy are to reduce pain and improve the function of your jaw joint. To this end, the therapist generally uses a combination of "hands-on" techniques. These might include massage, spray and stretch, and the use of various types of devices and equipment including heat, cold, and electrical stimulation.

TMJ sufferers are also urged to begin a program of regular exercise, stress management, proper nutrition, and correct posture, to prevent painful flare-ups. If you undergo physical therapy, you can expect to begin your program with three sessions a week. These visits will gradually decrease to once a week, and eventually culminate with a home program that only requires you to pass along periodic progress reports to your therapist. Most physical therapists work in physical therapy departments in hospitals or rehabilitation centers which explains why treatments are often so expensive.

Heat

For many TMJ sufferers, the benefits of heat are numerous. Such benefits include reduced inflammation, increased circulation, improved jaw function, and perhaps best of all, pain reduction. Heat also relieves muscle spasm which is responsible for the majority of TMJ problems.

The two main sources of heat used by many therapists are hydrocolators and ultrasound. A hydrocolator (a fluid-filled plastic pouch inserted into a fabric wrapper) provides moist heat which penetrates deeper than dry heat. Ultrasound, utilizing soundwaves, offers the deepest heat penetration but can pose a significant risk when used to treat TMJ problems. Too much ultrasound can cause irritation and jaw bone degeneration, after prolonged usage. There is some concern over the safety of ultrasound used directly on a surgical incision site or in a patient who has a TMJ implant.

Cold (Cryotherapy)

Cold, or cryotherapy, has the same end result as heat with the added benefit of numbing the painful area. The therapist may use a variety of ice packs or even give you an ice massage.

Heat and Cold

Used together, heat and cold can provide excellent benefits. Ice is generally used first to numb the painful area and increase the flow of fresh blood to the affected site. When ice is used before heat, the numbness simply helps you tolerate the heat better.

Electrical Stimulation

Several types of electrical stimulation are also used in physical therapy. One of the main ones is *Transcutaneous Electrical Nerve Stimulation* (TENS). During this procedure, a mild electric current is passed through tiny electrodes attached to various sites on the body. Proponents of TENS claim that it relieves discomfort by blocking the pain signal to the brain. Another theory is that it stimulates the body to produce more endorphins, or natural painkillers, stimulates blood flow, and relaxes muscles.

Some studies show that the use of TENS after surgery has reduced the need for post-op pain medication by as much as 90 percent. But others disagree, saying any alleged pain reduction is merely a placebo effect, since only anecdotal reports have been used as indications of TENS success. Unfortunately, such controversy is hard to resolve because TENS is a difficult type of treatment to study, due to the many technical and clinical variables involved in its use. There is little agreement among practitioners on amperage, frequency, duration, electrode placement, or mode of action (ADA, 1989).

Despite questions about its effectiveness, TENS has been

used by thousands of people for more than 20 years. Some people claim it allows them to lead more nearly normal lives. A small, battery-operated unit about the size of a calculator makes it convenient to use anywhere.

Myotherapy (Muscle Therapy)

During *myotherapy* a therapist applies pressure to trigger points, which relax muscle spasm and decrease, or relieve, pain. Some myotherapists utilize ice and exercise. A do-it-yourself approach is stressed.

Massage

Several different massage techniques are used by physical therapists, including *gentle massage, deep tissue* or *vigorous massage, myofascial release*, and *craniosacral massage*. In general, each technique is supposed to encourage the flow of blood and oxygen to different parts of the body in an attempt to restore mobility and relieve pain.

Myofascial release, for example, is based on the concept that pain and dysfunction are the result of muscle spasms and constrictions in the *fascia* (connective tissue) that covers the muscles, nerves, and bones. When a trained therapist exerts gentle but firm pressure on the jaw joint and parts of the face and neck, it supposedly releases the constriction, which reduces pain and increases range of joint motion.

Although not all massage methods are based on scientific fact, they do seem to provide some degree of pain relief and relaxation for many patients. When done properly, and used in combination with other treatments, you may find that massage definitely increases the range of motion and flexibility of your jaw joint. But, as with any treatment, the effects of massage will vary from one individual to another. You may get better, but you may also get worse.

Spray and Stretch

This physical therapy technique uses a cold spray, such as *flourimethane*, on the joint or muscle, causing a numbing effect. The therapist then gently stretches the muscles past the patient's restricted range of motion without causing discomfort or pain.

Range of Motion Exercises

Physical therapists often teach a series of gentle exercises that allow the muscles to relax and the range of motion to be increased.

Alternative Therapies

Many alternative therapies are becoming increasingly popular in the treatment of TMJ. These treatments include chiropractic, acupuncture, applied kinesiology, cranial manipulation, homeopathy, and nutrition therapies. You should know that they have never been scientifically proven to be safe and effective for the treatment of TMJ disorders and can make your condition worse.

Chapter 7

Implants: The Great American Medical Disaster

Since the early 1970s, approximately 60,000-80,000 Americans have received various types of artificial jaw joint implants (Fontenot, 1992). Sometimes surgeons replace just the disc with interpositional implants (IPIs); other times both the ball and the socket (condyle and fossa) are replaced with total joint prostheses. Some implant victims have undergone as many as 35 surgical procedures.

It is estimated that three to four times as many people have autogenous bone grafts, such as ribs, cartilage, or muscle flaps, or cadaver bones or tissues.

Vitek Implants

Perhaps the worst of the implants were the Proplast-Teflon implants manufactured by Vitek, Inc., of Houston. They were recalled between 1990 and 1991 due to their extremely high rate of failure. These include the IPI; the VK (Vitek Kent); and VK-I (Vitek Kent I). Since 1983, an estimated 25,000 people have received the IPIs, and no one knows for sure how many people have received the Vitek total joint prostheses.

Early reports in the 1970s claimed success with the Proplast-

Teflon implants, and in 1983, Vitek was given the green light from the FDA to market a precut disc. The company's president, Dr. Charles Homsy, merely had to convince the FDA that the device was substantially equivalent to Dow Corning's Silastic disc, marketed years earlier (see "Silastic Implants" below). Sales boomed.

In the early 1980s, Vitek developed the total joint known as the VK-I. It was changed in 1986 due to wear problems, and became known as the VK-II. At the 1986 meeting of the American Association of Oral and Maxillofacial Surgeons (AAOMS), several doctors reported catastrophic biomechanical failure of the IPI that caused a giant cell reaction, leading to bone resorption and pain. A summary of the literature from 1986 to 1991 reported a failure rate of 10-25 percent. In mid-1988, Vitek withdrew the IPIs from the market, citing escalating costs of litigation and product liability coverage. By 1992, a success rate of less than 20 percent was being reported.

Only after reports of failure began appearing in 1984 were animal studies conducted on dogs. The results were "essentially catastrophic," according to a 1990 deposition that Dr. Jack Kent, an oral surgeon involved in early research of the Vitek implant, gave in an Arizona court case against Vitek in Tucson. After just a few months, the Teflon layer was "completely worn" and Teflon particles had triggered bone erosion in the dogs.

In April 1989, the FDA reclassified the Vitek implants as Class III devices, meaning the manufacturer had to submit long-term safety and efficacy data in order to continue selling the products. Then in March 1990, Vitek issued a safety alert to oral surgeons. All doctors were not contacted, however, before Vitek declared bankruptcy in June and went out of business. Two companies, Oral Surgery Marketing, Inc. (OSMI) and Novamed, took over the sales of the implants at this point.

Vitek continued to market TMJ products and surgeons continued to use them, however. In October the FDA seized all the Vitek TMJ implants. Then in December, in an unprecedented action, the FDA issued its own safety alert to all members of AAOMS.

On January 7, 1991, the FDA recalled the disc implants and advised patients to have x-rays every six months as long as they had the implants in place. In March, Public Citizen Health Research Group petitioned the FDA to find patients with the Vitek implants to warn them of the serious risks and the need for immediate medical assessment. [Public Citizen is a nonprofit public interest group founded in 1971 by Ralph Nader. The Public Citizen Health Research Group, located in Washington, DC, was co-founded in 1971 by Ralph Nader and Dr. Sidney Wolfe, director.] Public Citizen was concerned that if patients weren't notified, they could suffer irreparable damage before they had any symptoms.

In September 1991, the FDA issued "Public Health Advisory on Vitek Proplast TMJ Implants" to oral and maxillofacial surgeons. A month later, an FDA press release announced the establishment of a notification program for patients with Vitek implants.

Silastic Implants

The history of jaw joint devices began with Dow Corning's introduction of Silastic (silicone rubber) Medical Grade Sheeting in the mid-60s. Short-term studies in the early 70s looked good. Surgeons learned to leave Silastic in just long enough for a smooth fibrous capsule to form around it. Then they removed the implant and the patient could function on the capsule.

Reports after one to five years, however, showed substantial problems, including ankylosis (permanent locking TM joint), arthritis, and lymph node swelling. One 1982 study warned doctors that particle migration meant they should be alerted to possible systemic reactions and foreign body synovitis, speeding failure (Gordon & Bullough, 1982).

A 1986 article reported fragmentation, perforation, and deterioration. Another stated: "Silicone may not be a totally inert material and its biomechanical properties are not ideal for use in the TMJ" (Dolwick & Audermorte, 1985). By the end of the 80s, enough failures had occurred for some researchers to call for strict limits on the use of Silastic.

By 1985, Dow Corning had a new design, the Wilkes device. A package insert recommending this product be used only temporarily was issued with each implant.

From Dow Corning's public documents and a review of the literature, it is clear they knew decades earlier what doctors found in 1985 — that Silastic is "intrinsically flawed as a biomaterial for long-term implantation into the human body" (Lappe, 1992).

As early as the 60s, they saw foreign body giant cell reaction and they knew it induced fibrosis and calcification. But even in the late 70s and early 80s, with the knowledge of the adverse effects of the wear particles, Dow Corning issued no adequate warning in the package insert and continued marketing it.

As late as 1989 there was not one long-term study of the use of Silastic in animals or humans. In 1991, when sheep studies were conducted, severe bony destruction and foreign body giant cell reaction were found. Finally, after 20 years of use, it was decided that Silastic wasn't appropriate for long-term use and that even short-term use is highly experimental (Bosanquet, Ishimaru, & Goss, 1991).

Many patients appear to be having the same kinds of difficulties with Silastic as those who have the Vitek implants. According to one radiologist, they appear to be failing in 10-15% of cases. Although the FDA has not recalled these implants, Dow Corning voluntarily removed them from the market in January 1993.

The TMJ implant device market has seen the development of several total joints consisting of various combinations of metal, acrylic, and plastic. Two major ones are those made by TMJ Implants, Inc., and Techmedica, Inc.

TMJ Implants, Inc.

TMJ Implants, Inc.'s total joint, commonly known as the Christensen device, has been around for 30 years. It's estimated that 3,500 of these devices have been sold since the late 80s. The founder of the company, Dr. Robert Christensen, claims 30 years of success, even though it appears that no long-term follow-up studies have been performed.

In spite of a lack of safety data, the company has continued to aggressively market their product in journals such as the *Journal of Oral and Maxillofacial Surgery*.

Techmedica, Inc.

Since 1989, Techmedica, Inc. has offered their total joints to a few select surgeons because they are custom devices made for the specific needs of each patient. As of June 1992, only six patients had Techmedica's custom-made implant for as long as three years. And although they appear to be doing okay in some patients, it is important to remember that the Vitek and Silastic implants looked good for the first few years. The concern is that they won't withstand long-term stresses of a load-bearing joint such as the TMJ.

Chapter 8

The Scandal Unfolds

When it comes to the TMJ implants, there is plenty of blame to go around. It is clear that governmental agencies, health care professionals, and device manufacturers have failed to protect the TMJ patients of this country.

To begin with, the American Dental Association has neglected to make TMJ a specialty with educational criteria and, even worse, has ignored the blatant quackery being practiced by American dentists. And the NIH has spent a mere .07% of its total budget on research of a disorder that affects approximately 30 million Americans. The majority of research they have funded has been to study the psychological aspect of TMJ, to the neglect of basic science.

The FDA has played a major role in the TMJ implant situation. Like the silicone-gel breast implants, jaw joint implants came on the market before the 1976 Medical Devices Amendment Act was passed requiring manufacturers to prove their devices are safe and effective. Because the TMJ implants were already on the market, no testing was required — even in animals.

TMJ implants were simply "grandfathered" in under the Act, which means that manufacturers only had to "prove" that their device were "substantially equivalent" to something already on the market.

Although the first failures of the Vitek implants were reported to the FDA in 1986, they dismissed them. Only in July 1988 — a month after Vitek pulled the product off the market — did the FDA conduct a comprehensive inspection of Vitek's plant.

The inspection turned up numerous violations. FDA officials claim Vitek wasn't relaying all of the problem reports it was receiving, as they were required to. On the other hand, the FDA was either unaware of, or failed to act on, several signs that something was seriously wrong. Such as Vitek's 1986 letter to surgeons, and a 1987 report from the U.S. Air Force concerning implant failures, severe pain, and bone erosion. Complaints from air bases prompted a notice to every branch of the armed services cautioning surgeons against using the IPI.

Although a special FDA panel had voted in April 1989 to classify all TMJ implants as Class III devices, this classification wasn't announced in the Federal Register until 3 years later! And then manufacturers were told they had 30 months to provide this safety data.

The FDA's role is to help "ensure the safety and effectiveness of drugs and medical devices," with primary authority over manufacturers. They clear new drugs and devices before they are marketed and monitor their performance, taking action when there are problems. Where TMJ implants are concerned, it is obvious that the FDA missed several opportunities to intervene and head off the IPI disaster.

Implant manufacturers are also responsible. They failed to conduct adequate safety studies on their products and continued to market them in the absence of long-term studies. And they discounted reports of adverse effects. What is Vitek's response? They claim the problems with their implants are exaggerated, and that they were targeted by the FDA to prove to Congress and health care advocates that it was beefing up regulation of the medical devices industry.

Dr. Charles Homsy, founder of Vitek, Inc., is now in "professional" exile in Switzerland. He blames just about everybody — except himself. He blames surgeons for putting his product in the wrong patients or for botching the procedure. Unbelievably, he still claims his product is perfectly safe. He blames Dr. Jack Kent, oral surgeon and researcher at Louisiana State University Medical Center, for gaps in testing. And, most shocking of all, he blames patients for not following postoperative instructions against opening their jaws wide or eating solid food until they are fully healed.

It is rather interesting to note that Dr. Kent owned 21,000 shares in Vitek. In early 1984, he wrote a letter to Dr. Homsy expressing his concern that, based on his experience with one of his patients, Vitek might have a "calamity of unbelievable proportions on our hands." This did not, however, deter him from continuing to publish articles praising the Vitek implants.

In general, oral surgeons claim they were unsuspecting victims who were taken advantage of by overzealous manufacturers. When you consider the high costs and considerable risks involved with TMJ implant surgery, you would certainly think surgeons have a responsibility to review and evaluate the evidence to support any procedure they are considering. It's unethical and irresponsible for doctors to say they assumed the implants had been tested. And it's a terrible disservice for oral surgery journals to advertise products that have not been clinically proven to be safe and effective.

Somehow, many surgeons overlooked information available to them in the medical literature that should have alerted them to serious problems with TMJ devices. As early as 1963, the orthopedic literature reported on the failure of Teflon used in hip prostheses, with fragmentation, giant cell reaction, and bony changes. "The orthopedists' experience could have predicted the long-term results described in the oral and maxillofacial surgery literature" (Wolford, 1992).

Even after they were instructed to notify their patients of the Vitek recall and risks, many oral surgeons have failed to do so. All members of the American Association of Oral and Maxillofacial Surgeons (AAOMS) received a copy of the FDA's "Safety Alert" concerning the Vitek implants. Later, in the "Public Health Advisory," they were asked to notify their patients, discuss the risks of device failure, and to continue to monitor them. In addition, they were told to encourage their patients to enroll in Medic Alert's International Implant Registry, and were given thirty days to complete Patient Notification Confirmation forms regarding the action they had taken.

A year later, only 312 patients had been registered with Medic Alert, and less than 200 notification forms had been received from surgeons. In August 1992, in their own "TMJ Implant Advisory," members of AAOMS were reminded that, "It is vitally important that you make concerted efforts to reach your TMJ implant patients," and to "be prepared to document your attempts to reach patients via phone logs, registered mail receipts, etc."

The TMJ Association has made numerous attempts to encourage AAOMS to issue formal advisory statements regarding implants. We are still waiting for an answer. The lack of serious effort put forth by AAOMS regarding this tragic disaster is appalling. Their blatant lack of accountability and compliance of FDA requirements is completely unacceptable.

But, AAOMS maintains that their foremost concern is for the "well-being" of patients. A recent editorial appearing in the *Journal of Oral & Maxillofacial Surgery* stated:

"What was done with good intent has now turned into a disastrous situation, with many patients worse off then ever before. To look for whom to blame, however, is a futile exercise. Rather, our responsibilities are now twofold: first, we need to seek ways to help these suffering patients return to a reasonably normal life; and second, we owe it to them and ourselves to see that a situation such as this never occurs again. Instead of pointing fingers at each other, patients and doctors need to join together in a common cause because all, in a sense, have been victims.... We all need to learn from these mistakes and find ways to prevent their occurrence in the future, but we also have a responsibility to face the immediate crisis. The media needs to make patients aware of potential problems, the patients need to seek consultation, and the practitioner needs to provide proper care. Working together rather than separately, we will not only resolve these issues, but hopefully will also find ways to prevent similar situations from ever occurring again" (Laskin, 1993).

Wouldn't it be wonderful to believe that the oral surgeons in this country will take responsibility for what has happened to the lives of so many implant victims? It remains to be seen what steps they will take to truly help their patients.

The Bottom Line

The roots of the implant disaster stem from a total lack of science where TMJ is concerned. TMJ is a disorder with no consensus on cause, diagnosis, or treatment. Doctors don't even agree on a definition. As a result, many patients have been ruined by unscientific and unproven treatments, the worst being the TMJ implants.

This deplorable situation didn't happen overnight. Many of these people with implants wouldn't have them if they had not first fallen victim to treatment after treatment that has no scientific basis whatsoever. They started off, in many cases, with the so-called "safe and irreversible" treatments such as splint therapy, equilibration, and steroid injections, and were led step by step to the point where they were convinced the only answer for them was surgery, and more surgery, and more surgery, until they finally ended up with implants.

The lives of many people with TMJ implants have been completely devastated. Some are seriously ill, unable to work, function daily, or lead normal, productive lives. They face a lifetime of chronic, unrelenting pain and disability. Some cannot obtain treatment — either because they can't find a doctor who will treat them, or because they have exhausted all their money and insurance. In some cases, they are unable to have failed implants removed. Many face multiple revision surgeries costing as much as $85,000, multiple removal surgeries, and continual follow-up care. Right now, there is no good alternative implant on the market. No matter what decisions they make, all options are costly.

Fixing this huge "medical mess" is going to take a lot of hard work from a lot of people. Combined expertise from scientists, medical as well as dental professionals, the FDA, the NIH, and device manufacturers, will be required. A first step might be admitting to the controversy and taking responsibility for the use of treatments that have ruined the lives of thousands of patients and make sure something like this never happens again. This will take a little honesty, and perhaps a setting aside of egos in the process. Too many people have lost too much to expect any less.

Implant Victims Turn to the Courts

An ever-increasing number of lawsuits, both class action and individual, are being filed against implant manufacturers. More than 3,000 suits have been filed against Vitek, but since the company is bankrupt, only a few thousand dollars, at best, have been awarded to patients.

Dupont, manufacturer of the Teflon part of the Vitek implant, is now being sued on the basis that they supplied Vitek with a defective material. Their response is that a sophisticated manufacturer such as Vitek should have been responsible for safety testing. Recent documents indicate that Dupont knew how its Teflon was being used and that, although it was inadequate, they continued to supply it to Vitek.

Dow Corning, manufacturer of the Silastic TMJ implant, is also involved in various lawsuits around the country. All these cases seek funds for future medical monitoring of patients with TMJ implants and recovery for injuries as a result of the defective devices. These suits claim that the implants have degenerated and the manufacturers are liable for selling defective and negligently made products.

Chapter 9

The Turning Point: Congress Intervenes

After three years of banging down doors, trying desperately to get someone to listen and do something about the implant tragedy, Terrie Cowley, President of The TMJ Association, Ltd., decided Congress was the only remaining alternative.

In early January 1992, she made the first contact with the Subcommittee on Human Resources & Intergovernmental Relations. This committee is responsible for overseeing the FDA and NIH and had only recently completed their investigation of the dangers of silicone-gel breast implants. Terrie begged them to look into the disastrous results of TMJ implants.

And this time, her relentless efforts really paid off. The result was the congressional hearing of June 4, 1992, entitled "Are FDA and NIH Ignoring the Dangers of TMJ (Jaw) Implants?" The purpose of the hearing was to review FDA and NIH policies on TMJ and jaw joint implants, as well as the safety and efficacy of current treatment modalities.

In his opening statement, Congressman Ted Weiss summed the situation up very well:

"As a result of the carelessness on the part of FDA, thousands of patients have suffered terribly from implants that never should have been allowed to be sold in the first place. Not only did the implants not work, not only did they cause unrelenting debilitating pain, they sometimes cause serious permanent damage that continues long after the implants are removed.... Not all patients have had pain and suffering because of their implants, but it may be that most eventually will. Most frightening of all, some of these implants are causing permanent damage to the skull, and the patients are not even aware that they are in danger" (Weiss, 1992).

Some of the objectives of the subcommittee were to determine:

1. Why has FDA failed to regulate TMJ implants?

2. Why has NIH failed to fund research on the safety of TMJ grafts or implants, or to determine the best possible treatment for the thousands of TMJ patients who have been damaged by their implants?

3. Most important, are millions of patients with many different kinds of implants put at risk while two federal health agencies pass the buck or drop it altogether? How often does FDA fail to require manufacturers to conduct research on their products, while NIH refuses to fund research on those same products because they believe it is FDA's responsibility? (Weiss, 1992)

Expert witnesses and representatives from the FDA and NIH provided some rather revealing testimony and made numerous recommendations. If carried out, it will certainly be a step in the right direction.

- In order to provide patients with safe and effective devices, it is imperative that scientists understand the biomechanics of both normal jaw joints and those that have been reconstructed.

- Research is desperately needed to determine the safety and effectiveness of devices. The consequences of failed implants, including the immune response, must be investigated. Acceptable alternatives must be found for patients whose implants have failed.

- To protect the public and avoid these problems in the future, improved regulatory mechanisms are needed so devices cannot be put on the market without proof of safety and effectiveness.

- Increased funding for research that will determine the outcomes of any type of surgery for TMJ disorders isnecessary to prevent future incidences.

- Patients must be informed about the risks associated with TMJ implants. This should be widely publicized through all media avenues.

- Effective ways to manage patients post-operatively must be identified through research and controlled studies. In order to develop methods of handling the severe, intractable pain experienced by many implant victims, the body's response to the giant cell reaction must be understood. Funding is needed for both the evaluation and treatment of patients with failed or failing implants.

- To evaluate treatment outcomes and provide long-term patient monitoring, a national center should be established. Patients should be encouraged to enroll in Medic Alert's International Implant Registry so the incidence and consequences of implant failure can be studied.

The highlight of the hearing was the testimony offered by three patients with TMJ implants. In obvious pain, they articulately and movingly described how TMJ implants had forever changed their lives. [For their complete testimonies, see the Appendix.]

Things Are Changing

A lot has been happening since the hearing. It is obvious that there is an increased awareness of temporomandibular joint disorders among patients, professionals, and governmental agencies. Finally, TMJ is being recognized as a legitimate disorder, not just something that affects "stressed-out" women. It appears that, just maybe, the scientific community is realizing the urgent need for research in order to develop safe and effective treatments for TMJ patients. And the government is being forced to do something about harmful devices.

FDA Finally Takes Action

Since the hearing, the following regulatory actions have been taken by the FDA.

- Products manufactured by **Oral Surgery Marketing, Inc. (OSMI), Novamed,** and **Vitek** have been removed from the market. The FDA recalled the implants made by Novamed, Inc., and Oral Surgery Marketing, Inc., two weeks prior to the hearing. These companies took over for Vitek in 1990 when Vitek went bankrupt.

- **TiMesh** has discontinued manufacture of the TMJ device.

- FDA conducted an inspection of **Dow Corning** in December 1992. In January of 1993, Dow discontinued the Silastic medical grade sheeting non-reinforced, Silastic medical grade sheeting reinforced, the Silastic medical grade sheeting non-reinforced extra firm and the Silastic TMJ Implant H.P., Wilkes Design. However, the FDA has yet to make a formal statement concerning the problems experienced by patients with Silastic TMJ implants.

- Presently, FDA is corresponding with **Osteomed** and **Techmedica** providing information which affords them the statutory requirements to make these devices legally available. The FDA has concluded that the Techmedica TMJ device requires FDA approval for marketing because it does not meet the requirements of a "custom device."

- The TMJ implants manufactured by TMJ Implants, Incorporated (Christensen TMJ) and The Temporomandibular Research Foundation (Morgan implant) have been found to be pre-amendment devices. That is, they were on the market before the 1976 Medical Device Amendment.

- The FDA has no safety and efficacy data on any TMJ products. However, they will require implant manufacturers to provide data concerning the safety and effectiveness of their devices in the future. An outside advisory panel has recomm-ended that all TMJ implants be placed into Class III, which means the manufacturers have to submit pre-market approval applications to the FDA with evidence of device safety and efficacy.

- Effective August 29, 1993, the Device Tracking Regulation requires manufacturers to establish systems to track jaw implants so patients who receive them can be notified if problems develop.

- Health professionals and patients can report problems with a device by calling 1-800-FDA-1088 and requesting a MedWatch reporting form.

Patients wanting copies of FDA documents should submit a written request to: Food & Drug Administration, Freedom of Information (HFI-35), 5600 Fisher's Lane, Rockville, MD 20857, and request any records not normally prepared for public distribution. They should include name, address, telephone number, and a statement of records being sought.

To receive the FDA's new publication entitled "TMJ Implants: A Consumer Information Update," write to the following address:

Food & Drug Administration, HFE-88
Office of Consumer Affairs
5600 Fishers Lane
Rockville, MD 20857

NIH Takes Problem Seriously

NIH has taken several long-overdue steps to address research and treatment needs.

- A meta-analysis, or literature analysis, was recently conducted to determine the scientific validity and efficacy of current treatments. According to the results of the meta-analysis, which was performed by Alexia Antczak of the Harvard School of Public Health, TMJ research studies are inadequate to determine whether any surgical treatments for TMJ disorders are safe.

  This may sound discouraging, but at least the NIH may be admitting to the fact that what we're dealing with is a complete lack of science. This is a big step and, hopefully, it's the first of many.

- The National Institute of Dental Research and the Office of Research on Women's Health are planning a study of various aspects of TMJ surgery and implants.

- To get an idea of just how far we've really come, read the NIDR's new informational brochure on TMJ. They have come a long way, too. To receive a copy, write to:

  National Institute of Dental Research
  9000 Rockville Pike
  Bldg. 31, Room 2C-35
  Bethesda, MD 20892

- By the time many people are reading this book, the very first International Workshop on Temporomandibular

Disorders and Related Pain Conditions will have been held in April 1994. According to NIDR, the primary goal is "To develop and prioritize research recommendations which can provide the basis for a Research Agenda on Temporomandibular Disorders, as well as for research on other pre-chronic and chronic craniofacial pain conditions." Specific goals are:

1. Developing research recommendations that will accelerate progress toward understanding the TMJ disorders and related pain conditions;

2. Assessing and summarizing the current state of knowledge on topics pertinent to the TMJ;

3. Assuring that the recommendations and assessment of current knowledge reflect a broad international perspective.

NIDR is providing leadership and support for the workshop, with co-sponsorship from the National Institute for Arthritis and Musculoskeletal and Skin Diseases (NIAMS) and the Agency for Health Care Policy and Research (AHCPR).

It is hoped that the workshop will develop consensus statements that will help form the basis for research recommendations for the following:

- How prevalent is TMJ?

- How is it distributed among the population (age, gender, race, etc.)?

- What causes TMJ disorders?

- What are the risk factors for developing TMJ, for example, oral habits, trauma, etc.?

- What impact does TMJ have on the individual in terms of function, psychological status, quality of life, work loss and disability, and cost?

- How does it impact on the family?
- What are the economic/financial impacts on the individual and society?
- Are existing diagnostic methods reliable and valid?
- Have current treatments been scientifically validated, for example, surgery, physical therapy, splints, drugs, behavioral and psychological therapy, and pain clinics?
- How can TMJ be prevented?
- How can chronic or recurrent pain be managed or prevented?
- What mechanisms are involved in joint and muscle pain?
- Are current surgical and non-surgical treatments effective? What are the short and long-term effects, for example, functionally, psychologically, and socially?
- What research methods can be used to determine the effectiveness and outcomes of various treatments?
- How cost effective is health care for the treatment of TMJ disorders?

Congress Urges More $s for TMJ Research

In April 1993, The TMJ Association testified before the Senate Appropriations Committee to plead for increased research funds for TMJ. We believe the fact that this disorder warranted a congressional hearing may have helped to ensure our success. The following report language, submitted by Senator Tom Harkin, was included in the Senate Appropriations bill for the 1994 National Institute of Dental Research (NIDR) budget.

"Temporomandibular disorder. Temporomandibular disorder [TMJ] is a common jaw disorder that can cause excruciating pain, difficulty in eating or talking, and other debilitating problems. Between 500,000 and 1 million new patients seek treatment for TMJ every year; 80 to 90 percent of whom are women. The Committee is aware that congressional investigations and clinical research have raised questions about the safety and effectiveness of certain treatments for TMJ, including implants and grafts, and urges NIDR to support research in this area."

This is an exciting success for all of us. When Congress "urges" a government agency such as the NIH to step up their support of research funds, it carries a lot of weight and generally gets done.

We've Come a Long Way!

When you think about where we were before the congressional hearing, it's encouraging to see so many things changing at last. Because of the congressional hearing and the work of The TMJ Association, the direction of TMJ research and treatment has been changed forever. At times, it's been a long, slow, and frustrating process. But according to Dr. Vivian Pinn, director of NIH's Office of Research on Women's Health, never has so much action been taken by NIH on a health disorder in such a short period of time. However, this is just the beginning.

There's Work to Be Done

If we could make a "wish list" that would incorporate solutions for many of the problems that led to this mess in the first place, it would probably look something like this:

- Basic scientific research must be carried out in order to determine the cause of TMJ.

- Current diagnostic methods must be evaluated and scientific guidelines developed that will accurately diagnose true TMJ problems.

- Available treatments need to be evaluated for safety and effectiveness. Sound treatments based on science must be developed that will lead to standards of care.

- Both the public as well as professionals who treat TMJ disorders need to be educated about the reality of the situation.

- There should be a specialty field for treating TMJ disorders that includes continuing education and professional certification.

- Dental schools should emphasize instruction on the scientific method. Dentists must understand how scientific knowledge is developed and verified. They need to know basic scientific principles. And they must know how to care for the problems of patients with TMJ disorders.

- Standards should be set for the sponsors of continuing education courses and seminars. The same goes for the speakers and course content.

- State laws should be strengthened so that dentists who practice unscientific and unproven treatments can be disciplined more quickly. Such disciplinary action should be made public.

- Medical professionals are needed to treat the numerous non-dental aspects of TMJ disorders, and should be trained to do so in medical school. For example, many people with TMJ problems have arthritis in their joints. And an estimated 80 percent have fibromyalgia. Professionals in these areas could provide invaluable expertise to this disorder.

- A huge national media campaign is needed to locate TMJ implant victims and inform them of the dangers associated with their implants and proper instructions about what to do.

- A more aggressive patient notification program is needed. The FDA should inform surgeons of problems with all TMJ implants and ensure that they, in turn, tell their patients.

- A national database of implant recipients should be established to track patients and for studying the physical, psychological, social, and financial damage caused as the result of the implants.

- Interaction among medical and dental professionals, the FDA, and various institutes of the NIH is needed to study implant patients for the extent of damage, both to the joint and systemically. Perhaps a way can be found to reverse or at least stop the destruction.

- Biomaterials research must be conducted that will lead to the development of safe and functional devices for patients who need replacement joints. It is important to also study tissues and other grafts used for TMJ reconstruction.

- Pain research is desperately needed if science is to learn how to manage and control the intractable, severe pain many implant victims are suffering. Programs to help these people cope and get on with their lives, or at least resume partially normal lives, would be extremely beneficial.

- The FDA should enforce stricter testing requirements of all diagnostic and treatment devices. More than 90 percent of applications submitted by device manufacturing companies are approved, which is not much incentive for companies to provide safety data on their devices.

- Solutions must be found for the insurance/financial problems faced by so many TMJ sufferers. Insurance companies should not be allowed to exclude scientifically validated treatments (both surgical and non-surgical) for jaw joint disorders. They should be covered on the same basis as any other diseased or dysfunctional joint in the body. Of particular urgency are people requiring implant removal, future surgeries, and lifelong follow-up care as the result of failed or failing TMJ implants.

- AAOMS should encourage its members to removed failed implants free of charge or at least on a sliding fee basis. They should also be encouraged to continue to provide necessary follow-up treatment for their patients, including helping them with pain management. (A little understanding and compassion wouldn't hurt either!)

- There is a desperate need for doctors to learn from their patients. After all, we are most qualified to provide input concerning the impact of TMJ and its effects on every aspect of our lives. As Dr. Harald Loe, former director of the NIDR, stated: "In the evaluation process we must not overlook the role of the patients themselves. For, as we know, in the end, the patients teach us" (Loe, 1993).

Chapter 10

The Story is Finally Told

Another positive result of the congressional hearing came a full year later with the first widespread national media exposure of the TMJ implant story. After years of trying to interest the news media in the burgeoning scandal, finally TMJ disorder exploded into the headlines in 1993. The August issue of *Woman's Day* featured a special report entitled "The TMJ Implant Disaster." Thanks to writer Barbara Deane, the TMJ implant story was finally in the news. It was followed closely by the August 31st issue of the *Wall Street Journal* featuring an article on the front page entitled "Medical Mess — Implants in Jaw Joint Fail, Leaving Patients in Pain and Disfigured," by Bruce Ingersoll and Rose Gutfeld. Then in November, *American Health* carried an article entitled "Jaws of Pain" by Cathy Sears.

In the television arena, ABC's "American Journal" and CBS's "Current Affair" both ran segments during the week of September 20th. And ABC's "20/20" covered the implant story on October 8th of 1993.

When the *Woman's Day* article hit the newsstands with "The TMJ Implant Disaster," The TMJ Association was flooded with calls and letters such as this one:

"You may not remember speaking with me about two weeks ago. I had the Vitek TMJ implants, which my oral surgeon never even told me were recalled by the FDA in 1991. He also failed to tell me my implants shattered into 15 pieces when he removed them back in 6/86. All these years, he told me my pain was psychosomatic!!! So, I continued with counseling and/or physical therapy, biofeedback, TENS, hypnosis, 13 surgeries, etc., etc., etc.

"I just cannot believe I've been so deceived all these years. The only way I learned of my condition was out of the *Woman's Day* article in 8/93. Then I confronted the oral surgeon.

"It's unbelievable what other victims and I are undergoing. To be lied to makes it even worse ... I think the only thing preventing me from taking my own life is somehow I feel I must try to help others. It's too late for me, but I do not want this to happen to one more person."

The vast majority of the people we heard from were implant victims. Many had undergone multiple surgeries, some with as many as six different materials and devices. And, with few exceptions, there were problems — sometimes serious ones. One patient summed the pain and suffering experienced by implant victims up very well: "It never goes away. I pray so hard for God to give me strength." And another said, "I just want my life back."

We heard stories that truly seemed to come from hell, as the lives of thousands of implant victims and their families have been devastated in every way imaginable — families torn apart, and left bankrupt, desperate, and without hope.

In conversations often lasting a few short minutes, people shared stories of pain, frustration, and fear — not just patients, but husbands, wives, mothers, fathers, friends — even children. And always, the inevitable cries for help.

We listened to voices filled with disbelief, then fear and anger, as many learned the truth for the first time. One woman said, "Not one professional told me what was going on. I didn't know what I had until I read the article." And another, virtually in shock, told us, "I haven't cried in a long time — maybe 10 years — and I cried like a baby when I read the article." When one patient asked why she wasn't notified about the Vitek implant recall, her doctor insisted he had been trying to find her. "Funny," she says, "the bill found me."

As appalling as the TMJ implant disaster is, it is even more appalling to hear how these people are being treated by the very professionals responsible for them. It's hard to believe the kinds of things doctors have the nerve to say to their patients: "It's your fault the implants failed," or "I don't know what went wrong. You're my only failure."

Frequently, patients are led to believe their pain and other medical problems are all in their heads and are referred to a shrink for psychological counseling. One 26-year-old patient was told: "You're a healthy young girl. Just learn to relax!" She says, "I would walk out of the doctor's office close to tears because I thought I was losing my mind." Some doctors tell their patients, "Don't worry ... there's no problem." Others abandon them — without a penny and in desperate need of having failed implants removed, further revision surgeries, and continual medical care. One patient was told, "There's nothing I can do. You're just going to have to learn to live with it."

With few exceptions, almost every letter and call we receive begins with "Thank God you're out there. Now I know I'm not alone." Many sufferers are desperate to talk with someone who's "been there" and doesn't think they are crazy. They need to know how to deal with their many emotions — anger, guilt, depression, and fear, as well as the many problems they encounter every day.

Over and over again, they say to us: "I thought I was the only one going through this," "I thought I was crazy," "I don't have anyone to talk to," and perhaps most frequently, "I feel so alone."

Well, the truth is you are not crazy and you are not alone. It's not all in your head and it most definitely isn't your fault if you haven't gotten better. Your pain is very real and there are thousands of others out there who are going through the same thing you are and they understand how you feel. They understand because they've been there.

Time and time again The TMJ Association is asked, "Has anybody else had this problem?" For many frequently thought they were the "only one." When they realized that thousands of others were going through the same thing and that somebody really understood, many broke down and sobbed uncontrollably. For them, their physical pain and emotional suffering were finally validated. They now have answers to questions they've had for years about their condition. Some now have the courage to stand up to their doctors and demand answers. "I became stronger when I realized I wasn't crazy," wrote one patient.

And many are angry and have turned their anger into positive action by doing what they can to change their situations and help others.

One patient, after a brief telephone conversation, later wrote:

"Thank you so much for giving of your time when I called today. You have given me hope that something will be done in the future. Just knowing that there is someone who really understands and is going through it herself gave me courage to keep fighting. I have support from my husband and daughter, but it's the understanding of someone who is going through this that gives me hope."

And another said, "Sometimes I wished I would never wake up in the morning. The article gave me a little glimmer of hope."

Hope — many now have hope for the first time, to go on and keep fighting. Sometimes, with too few answers to so many questions, the only hope we can offer is the truth, the assurance that an organization is out here fighting for you, and the realization that you can be intricately involved in future actions that influence your care and treatment. The TMJ Association is doing everything humanly possible to try and help you and to ensure something like the TMJ implant disaster never happens again.

Chapter 11

Frequently-Asked Implant Questions

I have a Vitek Implant. What's the problem?

According to studies, the implants are deteriorating — often without any clinical symptoms, yet perhaps with deadly consequences. By the time symptoms do appear, the damage can be well advanced and irreparable. Some people have experienced progressive bone degeneration in as little as one or two years, resulting in chronic excruciating pain, reduced jaw mobility, permanent loss of masticatory function, and in some cases, permanent hearing damage. There have also been reports of infection, facial deformities, vision problems, lymph node abnormalities, airway obstruction, and what the FDA calls "open communication to the brain" (skull perforations).

Various other health problems are being reported with a fairly high incidence, including systemic immune reactions such as fibromyalgia and the growth of non-malignant tumors in various parts of the body. At this time, the FDA and the medical community claim that the evidence that these illnesses are connected to the implants is not strong enough to draw a direct relationship; they claim more study is still needed.

What do I do if I have a Vitek implant?

If you have one of the Vitek TMJ implants, the Food & Drug Administration (FDA) has advised you to be examined by your doctor immediately and have a CAT scan or MRI. If the implant shows signs of deterioration, it should be removed as soon as possible — even if you have no symptoms — in order to minimize further damage. Patients with negative radiographs should be followed up carefully every six months as long as the implants are in place, to detect signs of breakdown. Contact your doctor if you are experiencing any of the following symptoms which may indicate that your implant is failing:

- pain radiating near the ear and/or severe headaches
- joint noise
- limited lower jaw movement and/or a change in the bite
- difficulty chewing
- nausea, dizziness, and/or vertigo
- ringing in the ears or hearing loss
- increased sensitivity in the head, neck, and shoulders

I had a Vitek implant removed last month. I'm okay now, aren't I?

Even if you have had your implant removed, the FDA is recommending that you be followed clinically to watch for possible residual damage. All the effects of these implants are not yet known, and there is no guarantee that the damage can be reversed.

I had an implant a couple of years ago, but I'm not sure what kind it is. How can I find out?

If you do not know what kind of implant you have, you may be able to find out by contacting your surgeon, the hospital where the surgery was performed, or your insurance company.

My doctor told me to enroll in an implant registry. What is he talking about?

The FDA is urging people who have Vitek implants, as well as those who have had them removed, to enroll in Medic Alert's International Implant Registry. You can do so simply by calling (800) 344-3226, 24 hours a day, 7 days a week. You will be asked to pay an initial enrollment fee of $25 and then $10 annually to compensate for the cost of maintaining your files. Enrollment in the registry enables you to receive up-to-date information on the implants as well as future information regarding any persisting symptoms and their treatment after removal. Also, you will be informed of any new devices and will receive continuing information in the event your doctor is no longer available. Finally, the registry will assist the FDA in locating patients and doctors if they need to be contacted in the future.

I have a Vitek implant, but so far have no problems. Do I need to have it removed?

Some doctors feel the implants should be removed no matter what because the failure rate is so high — almost 100%, and 50% fail within 3 years. Others feel they should be removed only if there is evidence of bone deterioration, you are experiencing symptoms, or both.

If your MRI shows damage and you are having symptoms, you will probably want to have it removed. If you have little, or minimal bone damage, and you're feeling okay (or at least not any worse than before the implants was put in), then you must decide whether to have it removed or not. Most patients seem to ultimately feel more comfortable after having their implants taken out, regardless of their condition. On the other hand, if it's been 8 or 10 years and you show minimal damage, you may feel reluctant to put yourself through another surgery. If you have no problems and decide to leave it in, you should know that you could later experience irreversible immune reaction that would undermine reconstructive surgery.

Okay, so I've decided to have my Vitek IPI removed. Now what?

It sounds discouraging, but treatments designed to replace an implant often fail. This is because of what is known as giant cell reaction. Whenever something artificial is put into the body, like a TMJ implant, the immune system sends out giant white cells in an attempt to destroy it or at least isolate it. Since these implants are made of non-organic material, the giant white cells remain around the implant, pumping out irritating chemicals in an attempt to eliminate it. Those chemicals dissolve tissue and bone, causing serious malformation. Even after removal of the implant, tiny particles are left that spread slowly throughout the body. The doctor can never get them all, no matter how many times he may try.

Unfortunately, right now there are no easy answers and very little consensus within the medical community. But you have several options. If you've had a lot of bone deterioration and are having trouble using your jaw and are in pain, many surgeons will recommend trying to rebuild all or part of the joint using autogenous grafting procedures, such as a rib, ear cartilage, or skin or muscle flap.

Other surgeons may recommend the use of a total joint prosthesis. There are two currently available (the Christensen and the Morgan), but there are no scientific, long-term studies proving either of them to be safe or effective. Some patients receive them and seem to do fairly well; others have horrendous problems with either the total joint itself or with continuing problems caused by having had Vitek in the first place.

Many patients go through a series of surgeries to try to reconstruct a joint that has been badly damaged by Vitek: removal of the implant, reconstruction with autogenous materials, and if that fails, a total joint, perhaps followed by other surgeries to clear out scar tissue or bony overgrowth which has formed. There simply is no evidence (scientific, anecdotal, or otherwise) that any of these surgical alternatives is safer or more effective than any other, or even better than doing nothing at all.

With minimal damage, sometimes surgeons will recommend removal, cleaning out the fragments and scar tissue, and not replacing it with anything, hoping that function might be maintained and pain kept to a minimum without additional reconstructive surgery. If the joint is functioning fairly well, this may be the safest and most conservative option. However, some patients find they develop scar tissue or occlusal changes which present a new set of problems. They may be manageable with conservative treatments, or your joint may fuse, making opening and moving your jaw more and more difficult.

When it comes right down to it, recommendations for patients with failed TMJ implants really depend on the doctors, what is available to them for implantation, and their individual bias or anecdotal information. Some patients who are in desperate need of implants believe all devices, even without safety and efficacy data, should be made available to them on a "buyer beware" basis. They point out that the FDA approved the material that destroyed their joints, and only too late has exercised its responsibility to "protect the public." Many patients express intense reservation and apprehension about the total joint they are considering for implantation. But, like they say, unlike breast implants, TMJ implants are necessary for survival and they are looking for the best of all evils. They are demanding explanations as to what the FDA is doing about this situation. And they deserve an answer.

Ultimately, many patients end up making decisions based on their own research, talking with other patients, consulting with many doctors, reading medical journals, and coming to a conclusion about what makes the most sense for them.

I was never contacted by my surgeon about the Vitek recall. Should I call him for an appointment?

If you feel comfortable doing so, you at least deserve an explanation as to why you weren't notified. If you choose not to return to the implanting surgeon, you can contact the nearest university dental school and see if they have experience dealing with Vitek patients. This could be at least a starting point for an initial consultation or referral for an MRI. You may be able to locate other patients who have the implants and find out if any of them have surgeons they are satisfied with.

Be sure any doctor you choose is very familiar with the history and problems associated with these implants. Don't be afraid to ask some tough questions and expect some honest answers. Questions include:

- How many implants have you put in?
- When did you stop using them?
- What problems have you seen?
- How do you feel about removal?
- How many have you removed?
- What treatment do you suggest following removal?

- On what basis do you make these treatment recommendations?

- Do you have any financial interest in any of these options or other specialists you refer to me?

Important: Ask for names of other patients who have been treated similarly to what your doctor is proposing for you. Call them and find out how they're doing.

The FDA recommends you find out how long a device has been on the market, and the name, manufacturer, model number, and lot number. Also, you should know if the labeling indicates it is a temporary or permanent device. If temporary, how long should it stay in? Be sure to find out about possible complications and advantages, and any alternatives available to you.

I've decided to have my implant removed. Will my insurance pay for it?

Many patients automatically believe that the government or manufacturer will pay the costs associated with removal. After all, these materials have been marked as hazardous to your health by the FDA and most medical professionals, so it's a medical necessity to have them removed.

Unfortunately, nothing could be farther from the truth. Not only will the cost of the removal surgery and subsequent treatment be yours and/or your insurance company's responsibility, some companies are refusing coverage for even the removal on the grounds that TMJ is a dental condition. Or, some policies have a cap on coverage and it may not be enough to cover even the surgeon's bill. Some pay so little that the health care providers may be reluctant to accept you as a patient. Still others are very good and will immediately approve removal and subsequent treatments.

There are a few scattered surgeons across the country who

have removed the implants free of charge, but hospitals will very rarely waive their fees. Other surgeons may reduce their usual cost and a few may go to bat for you in trying to help convince your insurance company that the consequences of leaving the implants in will result in much more major medical expense to the company in the future than if the insurance approved the removal now, regardless of whether they classified TMJ as dental or not.

My doctor has refused to treat me. What should I do?

If any surgeon dismisses your complaints or won't treat you, the FDA recommends that you write to your state dental association or AAOMS. The experience of patients who have tried this avenue suggests, however, that you may not get much help.

One of the most serious and frightening results of this whole disaster is the complete breakdown of communication between patients and doctors. Some doctors have abandoned their patients, at first by not returning their phone calls, and eventually refusing to treat them at all.

Implant patients who are steadily getting worse want to be fixed, and justifiably so. Their doctors have no solutions and, in many cases, are afraid of being sued. Unfortunately, at this point, there are no viable alternatives for patients in this situation. All we can hope is that, with proper research, ethical medical professionals will find ways to improve the quality of life of TMJ implant victims.

I have so much pain that I can't stand it without a lot of heavy medication. But I'm afraid of becoming an addict and my doctor says he won't write me prescriptions forever. What do I do?

Many implant victims have undergone multiple (as many as 35) surgical procedures that lead to chronic, debilitating pain.

Some are in such horrendous pain they can't stand it without medication. Yet, in many instances, their doctors are refusing to give them what they need to function, partly because of state reporting requirements, but also because they may discount the amount of pain their patients are suffering. They often suggest that you are simply a drug addict.

If you are in so much pain you are suicidal, you probably feel that becoming dependent onsomething that makes life a little more bearable or helps you get through another day, is secondary. Addiction is a separate medical issue that can be dealt with after a way is found to treat or deal with the pain.

Many patients believe drugs should be prescribed more freely when needed. Just knowing that relief is available actually decreases the actual use, as opposed to having to go to doctors to "scrounge" for medication.

Important: If you are taking any type of long-term medications, you should be monitored for signs of depression or adverse reactions caused by the medication and not the pain. And remember to always inform your doctors and anesthesiologists before undergoing any kind of anesthesia — general, "light sleep," or local. It can be fatal if the anesthesiologist doesn't make an adjustment in the amount of anesthesia used during surgery.

I became pregnant last month and still have a Vitek disc in my right jaw joint. Is there anything to worry about?

At this point, we don't really know. If you have questions, contact Children Afflicted by Toxic Substances (CATS), a new non-profit foundation, at (800) CATS 199, or write to them at the address below:

CATS
60 Oser Ave., Suite 1
Hauppaugue, NY 11788

I have a Silastic TMJ implant. Is there anything to worry about?

The FDA is receiving an increasing number of patient reports of failure and problems with the Silastic implants. These include chronic pain, bone and tissue deterioration, various blood disorders, and immune inflammatory responses.

If you are having problems, you should contact your oral surgeon because there is a possibility the implants may need to be removed. If you are not currently experiencing any symptoms, you should still be monitored closely by your oral surgeon because the implants, many of which were intended for short-term use only, can disintegrate over longer periods of time. According to the FDA, problems seem to be related to length of time the implant is in place, the anatomical configuration of the patient's joint, and how force is applied in the jaw area.

A Final Note

If you have a Vitek, Silastic, or any other type of TMJ implant and would like to voice your concerns, write to:

Dr. Donna Shalala, Secretary
Department of Health & Human Services
200 Independence Ave. SW
Washington, DC 20201

Dr. David A. Kessler, Commissioner
Food & Drug Administration
5600 Fisher's Lane
Rockville, MD 20857

Congressman Edolphus Towns
Committee on Government Operations
Subcommittee on Human Resources &
  Intergovernmental Relations
B-372 Rayburn Building
U.S. House of Representatives
Washington, DC 20515

Dr. Harold Varmus, Director
National Institutes of Health
9000 Rockville Pike
Bethesda, MD 20892

President
American Association of Oral & Maxillofacial Surgeons
9700 W. Bryn Mawr Ave.
Rosemont, IL 60018-5701

President
American Dental Association
211 E. Chicago Ave.
Chicago, IL 60611-2678

Chapter 12

Helping Yourself

If you think you may have a jaw joint disorder, start by seeing a medical doctor to rule out other problems that may mimic TMJ, such as sinusitis, an ear infection, migraine headaches, an abscessed tooth, or a tumor.

One question you should ask yourself, particularly if your TMJ symptoms have started suddenly is, "Has anything changed in my life recently that could possibly be causing my symptoms?" Some things to consider are changes in posture, talking on the telephone excessively, carrying a heavy shoulder bag, chewing gum, changing your mattress, pillow, or sleeping position, standing or sitting more than usual, typing for long periods of time, or lifting a heavy object, including your child. Try changing any of these situations that apply to you and observe what happens. Even stress factors, such as a new job or a divorce, can possibly create TMJ trouble because they may lead to muscle spasm.

Many people with TMJ disorders have minor problems that can be alleviated with conservative treatment or no treatment at all. Often, the problem goes away, so don't become discouraged and give up too quickly. If you are in the early stages of TMJ, you may find relief with some or all of the following self-help treatments.

Moist Heat

Heat can sometimes help reduce inflammation, muscle spasm, and pain. It may also improve the function of your jaw joint. Use a heat pack or hot water bottle with a warm, wet towel wrapped around it, being careful not to burn yourself. **Caution:** People with circulatory problems should not use heat without consulting a doctor first. Also, children and the elderly should be supervised while using any kind of heat source.

Ice

Ice has the same effect as heat and also increases blood flow, promotes healing, relaxes muscles, and has a pain-numbing effect. If you use an ice pack, be sure to wrap it in a clean cloth and don't leave it on for more than 10-15 minutes since you can damage your skin. For an ice massage, you can freeze water in a styrofoam cup with a popsicle stick in the end and then tear away the cup and use the stick as a handle. When used directly, ice can freeze the skin quickly, so it should not be used for longer than 5-10 minutes. For this reason, people with impaired circulation or skin sensation should not use a cold pack at all.

(Note: Try alternating between ice and heat — 10 minutes of ice followed by 10 minutes of heat, for an hour or so.)

Heat and Cold - Products for Pain Relief

There are many excellent products on the market that provide a convenient source of heat and/or cold. Some of the ones most appropriate for TMJ are reviewed below.

Heat Comfort Reusable Hot Pack - Made by 3M, this convenient hot pack can be heated either in the microwave or on top of the stove. Whichever method you choose, it only takes a few minutes. Its flexibility allows you to mold it comfortably to your face, back of the neck, and shoulders — all common sources of pain for TMJ sufferers. Available in most drug stores; Cost is $5.00.

Cold Comfort Reusable Cold Pack - 3M's gel-filled cold pack comes with a cloth-like protective cover. It must be kept in the freezer for approximately 2 hours to reach the coldest possible temperature. Recommended use is 20 minutes on, 20 minutes off. For tension headaches or migraines, you can apply the cold pack to the base of the neck. It is fairly pliable, even when frozen, and can also be used as a source of heat by boiling it as you would the hot pack. Available in most drug stores; Cost is $5.00.

Elasto-Gel Hot/Cold Packs - Southwest Technologies has a variety of products that can be used as sources of both moist heat and cold. They come in more than 40 sizes so there is one for almost every part of the body. Of particular interest to TMJ sufferers is the TMJ Wrap, for approximately $35. Also, they have several cervical support pillows and cervical collars for the neck. When used for heat, the Elasto-Gel products take less than 3 minutes to warm and retain the temperature for 20-40 minutes. If you want cold instead, they will cool in the freezer in 15 minutes. Either way, they stay soft and flexible. Costs range from $10 to $60. For more information, call (800) 247-9951.

Cool Dana/Warm-Upz - These two products, one for cold and the other for heat, can either be tied around your face, (over both joints, the top of your head and your chin) or around your head like a sweatband. They are flexible, comfortable, and maintain their temperature longer than regular ice or heat packs. They are colorful, so you won't look sick when you wear them. Cost is $10 + $3.95 shipping and handling, available from the TMJ Implant Patient Support Network by calling (504) 866-2111.

Thermophore Hot Pack - This electric hot pack produces

moist heat by drawing moisture from humidity in the air. You control the temperature. Several sizes are available with a petite size for TMJ sufferers which costs $45.95. For more information, call Battle Creek Equipment Co. at (616) 962-6181.

Self-Massage

Jaw/Face: To relax sore jaw and facial muscles, slowly open and close the mouth as wide as comfortably possible. Repeat five times. Then move the jaw slowly and gently from side to side five times. Using your fingertips, lightly massage the area over the jaw joints. Then clench and unclench your teeth three times.

Head: Gently massage the temples with the fingertips for 30 seconds using a slow circular motion. Massage scalp with fingertips with deep, slow strokes. Press the palm of your hand against your forehead and count to ten. Repeat on the sides and back of the head.

Neck: To loosen tight, painful neck muscles, turn your head slowly to the right and hold for five seconds. Return to the center. Do five times. Repeat to the left side. Tilt your left ear down toward the left shoulder and count to ten. Return to the center. Do five times. Repeat, tilting to the right side five times. Lower your chin down to your chest and hold for five seconds. Return to the center. Repeat five times. Using your hands, knead the muscles between your neck and shoulder.

Shoulders: Stand and raise shoulders as high as possible, trying to touch your ears, for five seconds. Relax. Do five times. Roll shoulders in complete circles forward and backward, five times in each direction.

Note: For hard-to-reach areas, a shower massager or hand-held electric massager works well.

Overall Health

Anyone who suffers with chronic pain of any type certainly does not need other health problems. Chronic pain causes stress, and stress lowers the body's resistance to disease. Fortunately, 80 to 90 percent of the viruses and bacteria that enter the body never make us sick. This is true because of the immune system which has two jobs: (1) it keeps bacteria and viruses from getting into the body in the first place; and (2) it kills the ones that do manage to get in.

Our lifestyles and environments dramatically affect the immune system's efficiency. Taking responsibility for your health through proper diet, exercise, rest, and stress management bolsters your immune system. They are all important factors in coping with illness of any kind.

Nutrition

Proper nutrition is also important to your overall health, especially the healing process. TMJ sufferers often have difficulty chewing because of pain or limited jaw function. But you can still get adequate nutrition. Most foods can be blended to a texture you can handle. They may be a little different than what you are normally used to, but you may be surprised just how good they can taste.

Soft Diet

Temporarily eating soft or blended foods may help by allowing the jaws and surrounding muscles to rest. Especially avoid hard, crunchy, or chewy foods, or foods that require you to open your mouth wide such as an apple or corn on the cob. (Don't chew gum!)

Exercise

Physical movement can be invigorating and refreshing. During exercise, your body produces more endorphins that decrease pain and help you relax. Walk, ride a bicycle, or swim. Even dancing feels great, especially to your favorite music. (This is really fun if you sing and act crazy.)

If you can't do anything very strenuous, try gentle stretching exercises, particularly of the upper body. Go slowly at first and gradually increase repetitions as you begin to limber up. Stretching exercises strengthen muscles and improve flexibility and joint function. In addition, exercise makes you feel better all over, increasing your energy level, and improving the way you feel about yourself.

Important Reminder: It's a good idea to have a complete physical before starting a new exercise program.

Watch Your Mouth

Gentle jaw exercises, such as slowly opening and closing your mouth as wide as comfortably possible, and moving your lower jaw from side to side, can improve mobility. Avoid anything that requires you to open your mouth very far, such as wide yawning or lengthy dental appointments. When you do go to the dentist, ask him to let you stop and close your mouth every 10 minutes or so to prevent muscle spasm and pain.

Make Your Own Splint

Some patients seem to have some luck with making their own splints. You can go to an athletic supply store and buy a mouth guard for $2 or $3. It comes with very clear instructions on how to custom fit it to your mouth.

Harmful Habits

Many doctors feel it is important for patients to recognize harmful habits and change them. One technique that has been suggested is known as habit reversal which teaches the patient to replace a harmful habit with its opposite. For example, if you catch yourself clenching your teeth, concentrate on keeping them apart for 30 seconds at a time.

Over-the-Counter Analgesics

You may have to experiment with several pain killers until you find the one that works best for you. Acetaminophen, such as Tylenol, helps some people, whereas others find relief with aspirin or Ibuprofen. (Hint: To lessen stomach irritation, try taking 20-30 minutes after a meal.) As with prescription drugs, check with your physician before taking any type of medication. [See Chapter 13 for more information on drugs.]

Join A Support Group

Support groups provide the opportunity for people with TMJ (and their families) to share information, and also offer encouragement and hope. Perhaps most importantly, you will be able to talk with other people who really understand what you're going through. If you can't find a TMJ support group in your area, look for a chronic pain support group or consider starting one yourself. [For more information on support groups, see Chapter 18.]

Chapter 13

Drugs and Tips for Safe Use

Carol is on so much heavy medication that she's afraid to go to sleep at night because when she wakes up she'll be going through severe withdrawal. She has really lost all hope and, as she told me recently, only wants to die.

The worst part of my TMJ nightmare began with a prescription for Xanax. The orthodontist who prescribed it told me to take it before bedtime. He said I wouldn't grind my teeth in my sleep and would wake up in the morning, free of pain. Because I'm very sensitive to most drugs, I questioned him carefully about side effects and the potential for addiction. He assured me Xanax was nothing more than a mild muscle relaxer and that I had nothing to worry about. Little did I know that I was in for the most frightening time of my entire life.

To make a long story short, I took Xanax as directed for almost two weeks before I started having unpleasant side effects. After talking with my pharmacist, I abruptly stopped taking it. Within three days I found myself in the emergency room with chest pains, feeling like I couldn't breathe, and pretty sure I was going to fly apart. After undergoing several tests, the internist I saw told me I was suffering drug withdrawal. He sent me home with directions about how to gradually get off the Xanax and how to use a paper bag whenever I began to hyperventilate.

For almost three months I went through hell, and was so scared most of the time that I couldn't be left alone. But with the support of my family and self-hypnosis, I finally quit cold turkey. Sometimes I felt like I would do anything for "just one little pill," but I knew I couldn't take another one because I would have to start all over again. If I had known how long it was going to take, I'm not sure I could have gone through it. (I later learned that it can be dangerous to withdraw from a drug such as Xanax without medical supervision.)

I was extremely angry that this had happened to me because it was all so unnecessary. I started doing a little research of my own to find out more about Xanax. To my surprise, I learned that Xanax belongs to the benzodiazepine anti-anxiety drug group. Since the dependency rating is high, it is usually not given for more than two weeks. Also, anyone taking the drug should talk to a doctor before stopping it because abrupt cessation can lead to withdrawal symptoms.

Why didn't anyone tell me this? Certainly doctors should have a responsibility to caution their patients about the possible side effects of the drugs they prescribe, including information about interactions with other drugs, and tell them how to stop taking a drug safely. You would at least expect this information from your pharmacist. Unfortunately, patients are not given accurate information, or enough information. So, we take drugs without this knowledge, and the results can be devastating.

I learned the hard way. My experience with drug addiction and withdrawal taught me to learn as much as I possibly can about any drug — either prescription or over-the-counter — that I take for any reason. In this chapter, I have assembled some information about drugs commonly used to treat TMJ disorders. More importantly, there are tips that will ensure that you take your medication as safely and effectively as possible.

Common Drugs for TMJ Treatment

During the initial phase of treatment, some doctors prescribe anti-inflammatory drugs, like aspirin, or sometimes ibuprofen to relieve pain. Still others prescribe tranquilizers such as Valium, and muscle relaxers such as Flexeril. Many of these drugs have unpleasant side effects and can be addictive. The NIDR recommends short-term use of muscle-relaxing and anti-inflammatory drugs when necessary (NIDR, 1993).

Non-Narcotic (Mild) Analgesics

There are several non-narcotic pain killers available over the counter.

Acetaminophen is effective for pain relief, except in cases of inflammation. It is considered to be one of the safest of all analgesics and is not apt to upset the stomach the way aspirin or ibuprofen does. Overdoses can be fatal, however, so acetaminophen is used with caution for people with kidney or liver disease. Alcohol may increase its toxic potential.

Ibuprofen is effective for pain and is also an anti-inflammatory. Common over-the-counter forms of ibuprofen are Motrin and Advil. One drawback of the drug is that it can cause stomach upset. Patients with ulcers or other stomach problems probably shouldn't use it.

Aspirin is especially effective for inflammation and swelling. It is often found in combination with other substances in a variety of medicines. A main drawback is its potential for stomach irritation, but this can be reduced by taking it after a meal. Some aspirin preparations like Bufferin are coated, or buffered, to avoid stomach irritation. But you may also take an antacid or a glass of milk for the same effect. Aspirin probably shouldn't be used by people with ulcers or other stomach problems or those who have a disorder that affects the blood's clotting function. Children under 18 shouldn't take aspirin either, because of the risk of Reye's Syndrome.

Other Nonsteroidal Anti-Inflammatory Drugs (NSAIDS)

Feldene, Voltarin, and Lodine, are frequently used for more severe pain. They can irritate the stomach lining, however, and are not usually given to people with stomach ulcers.

Narcotics, or Opioids

These are the most powerful and effective analgesics. They work by actually blocking pain signals to the brain. Some of the most common ones are morphine, methadone, and codeine. Side effects include constipation, drowsiness, confusion, and nausea. Withdrawal can occur if the drug is stopped suddenly. Narcotics become less effective over time, and should be started slowly and increased very gradually. They are controlled drugs because they can produce euphoria which can lead to abuse and addiction.

Hypnotics, or Sleeping Drugs

Hypnotics, or sleeping drugs, may be prescribed for insomnia due to pain, anxiety, or depression. Benzodiazepines are the main class of these drugs, and have fewer side effects than others (barbiturates, for example). Side effects include dizziness, drowsiness, and unsteadiness. If taken regularly for more than a few weeks, psychological and physical dependence may result. Abrupt withdrawal may produce sleeplessness, nightmares, anxiety, seizures, and hallucinations. Since their effect diminishes with time, stronger doses are usually required.

Antidepressants

A variety of drugs, like Elavil, are used to treat depression. In recent years, however, their use has become common to treat chronic pain such as fibromyalgia and arthritis. Much smaller doses are needed for pain than for depression. The two main kinds are tricyclics and monoamine oxidase inhibitors (MAOs). Improved sleep is immediate, but help for depression may take 10-14 days, and maybe 6-8 weeks for the full anti-depressant effect to be felt. **Warning**: Overdose of either drug is dangerous and may even be fatal. Side effects include drowsiness, dry mouth, blurred vision, and difficulty urinating.

Anti-Anxiety Drugs (Minor Tranquilizers)

These drugs are used to alleviate persistent feelings of nervousness and tension caused by stress or other psychological problems. Most commonly used are benzodiazepines, such as Lorazepam, Diazepam, and Clonazepam. Beta blockers, like Propranolol, are used less frequently. Side effects of benzodiazepines include drowsiness, apathy, muscle relaxation, and forgetfulness. Since patients become tolerant to their effects, they are usually effective only for a few weeks. Physical and psychological dependency are possible after prolonged use and withdrawal symptoms may occur if you stop taking them suddenly.

Tips for Safe Drug Use

According to studies, more than 50% of people take their prescription drugs incorrectly. This can be extremely dangerous. The following suggestions will help to ensure that you take prescribed medications safely.

- It is imperative that you know the benefits and risks of any drug you are taking. Find out how long it's been on the market and its track record in terms of safety.

- Ask about side effects and anything you can do to minimize them. Find out if the drug will affect any other health problems you have, such as high blood pressure.

- Tell your doctor about any allergies, especially allergies to drugs. Make sure this information is included in your medical record. (Allergic individuals are four times more prone to drug reactions than those who are free of allergy.)

- Ask if there are any special precautions to observe: avoidance of certain foods, alcohol, exposure to sun, other drugs, driving or other hazardous activities.

- Find out how long the drug can be taken safely. Ask your doctor if it is physically and/or psychologically addictive. Also, is it safe to stop the drug abruptly, or should you taper off gradually to avoid withdrawal symptoms?

- Ask your doctor if there is a generic equivalent for the drug. Generics are usually less expensive.

- Ask your physician for written information about the drug prescribed. You will not remember all of the information and instructions that you have been given verbally.

- Be sure you know the name (and correct spelling) of the drug(s) you are taking — both the brand name and the generic name. Be careful of drug names that look alike or sound alike, for example, Xanax and Zantac. Mistaking one drug for the other can be extremely dangerous. A prescription drug can easily be confused when given by telephone. Specifying the name of the disorder on the prescription will alert you and the pharmacist of a mistake.

- Be sure to read the warning labels on both the container and label. These are important reminders regarding the proper use of the drug. They provide important precautions that improve the effectiveness of your medication.

- Follow all instructions carefully and completely. Do not change the dose or timing of any drug without the advice of your physician. If the prescription says four times a day, does it mean four times during the time you are awake, or four times in 24 hours?

- Be sure you know exactly how to take the drug. For example, should you take it on a full stomach, or 1-2 hours before a meal? Should it be taken with water, milk, food, or mixed with something?

- Find out how medication should be stored. Most drugs are kept in cool, dry places, away from direct sunlight and heat, but some need to be refrigerated. And always make sure your medications are closed tightly.

- Make sure you know what to do if you miss a dose. Do you double up on the next one? Also find out what to expect if you exceed the recommended dosage.

- Contact your doctor immediately if you feel a drug is causing adverse effects.

- Notify your doctor if you develop any new symptoms after you start taking the drug(s) prescribed.

- If you are taking medications prescribed by more than one doctor, check the generic names of all prescriptions to be sure you are not taking duplicate drugs with different brand names. This could cause serious overdosage.

- Never take drugs prescribed for someone else. Also, don't offer drugs prescribed for you to anyone else.

- Periodically, check to make sure the drugs you take have not expired. The effects of most drugs diminish with time, so discard outdated drugs.

- Do not take any more medicines than absolutely necessary. (The greater number of drugs taken simultaneously, the greater the likelihood of adverse effects.)

- Never take a drug in the dark. Make sure you have adequate light to be certain you are taking the drug intended. It is best not to keep drugs on a bedside table unless they are for emergency use (such as nitroglycerin).

- Do not take any drug (prescription or nonprescription) while pregnant or nursing an infant until you talk to your doctor. If you become pregnant while taking medication, notify your doctor immediately.

- Keep track of any drugs to which you become allergic or experience an adverse reaction. (This should be done for each member of the family.)

- Make sure you keep follow-up appointments with your physician; it is important to closely monitor many drugs.

- Whenever you go to another doctor, be sure to tell him about all medications you are taking — both prescription and nonprescription.

- When you get a refill, make sure it's identical to the drug in your original supply. If it is not the same, ask your pharmacist to explain the difference. (Generic drug products from different manufacturers often vary in size, shape, color, etc.)

- If possible, use the same drug store and pharmacist. Most pharmacists utilize a computer system that records and analyzes each patient's drug history. This helps to prevent serious allergic reactions and drug interactions. Be sure your pharmacist is aware of all drugs you are taking.

- Inform your anesthesiologist and doctor of all drugs you are taking, prior to any surgery.

- To prevent accidental poisoning, store all drugs to be retained for intermittent use out of the reach of children.

- **REMEMBER**: Never be afraid to ask your pharmacist and/or doctor questions about your medications. After all, that's what they are for! It may help to write down your questions so you don't forget them. If you do not clearly understand instructions, call your doctor or pharmacist.

There are several excellent books available that will help you learn all about the drugs that have been prescribed for you. They may vary somewhat, but most provide information on dosage, instructions for taking them, side effects, drug interactions, and specific warnings.

Chapter 14

Mind Over Body

Evidence is mounting that the mind has a powerful role in healing the body. In fact, researchers in the relatively new field of psychoneuroimmunology (the study of how our minds affect our immune systems) have found what may turn out to be a powerful link between attitude and health. Thousands of clinics, hospitals, and private practitioners are providing training in how to use your mind, attitudes, and lifestyle to influence your health and quell pain.

Although not completely understood, it is well known that chronic psychological stress affects the immune system and its ability to fight disease. When the mind controls the body, stress is reduced and the immune system is bolstered.

The placebo effect — in which a doctor gives a patient a worthless treatment and the patient believes it is a cure and shows improvement — is well documented and works for a significant number of patients. For example, some doctors suggest to their patients that when they wake up from general anesthesia they will feel very little pain. Often they need much less medication than they would have if the suggestion had not been made.

Relaxation Techniques

Relaxation techniques can play a major role in your overall care by lowering your heart rate, blood pressure, and levels of stress hormones. Visualization (or guided imagery) in which you picture in your mind a pleasant memory and imagine yourself there, helps some patients correct their breathing and reduce muscle tension.

With progressive relaxation, you systematically relax various groups of muscles, beginning with your toes and working towards your head. This technique can be particularly useful when you have to endure lengthy x-rays or other procedures that are time-consuming or unpleasant. Other relaxation methods include slow, deep breathing, and alternately tensing and relaxing your muscles.

There's no question about it. When you're tense, your pain is worse. If you can learn to relax, your pain may become more tolerable. You might consider taking a course in stress management or read a book about relaxation techniques. Or buy one of the many relaxation tapes that are available. I have had great success with the one that contains the sounds of the ocean. Even on my worst days, when I listen to the waves and seagulls, I am able to visualize myself on a calm, quiet beach, and I can actually feel the sun on my skin and smell the suntan lotion. It is easier to fall asleep when I am this relaxed — in spite of my pain.

There are many relaxation techniques for coping with pain and the stormy emotions that come with it. Many are really distraction techniques, in which you focus on something other than your pain. It is similar to a pregnant woman going through natural childbirth, concentrating intently on her breathing, massage, and a focal point.

You may have tried some of these previously without even realizing that you were using your mind to control your body.

They are all safe, and some can really be so simple and work so well that it is almost unbelievable at times. You may have to experiment a little to see which ones work for you. Sometimes, a combination of methods may work best.

Hypnosis

Most people can be hypnotized, though some make better candidates than others. Like anything, self-hypnosis takes practice. Depending on the depth of the trance you are able to achieve (light, medium, or deep), it is even possible to undergo major surgery with no anesthesia. Not everyone can do this, but I think just about everyone can achieve some degree of control, or at least relaxation, through self-hypnosis. More and more doctors are recognizing that hypnosis can reduce pain and promote healing. Why not try it yourself? Here's how:

- Locate your pain and begin moving it down through your body, slowly, gradually, letting the pain flow out of your body and into the chair, the earth, the air.

- Think about whatever relieves your pain the most. It might be a warm bath, a pill, being quiet in a dark room, or a brisk walk through the park. Since you have the memory of pain relief built into your mental computer, simply reproduce that experience and let it relieve your pain. Hook yourself into your memory bank and play back the tape that previously rid you of unwelcome pain. A quick technique here to get you started is to remember your last shot of Novocain from the dentist. Reproduce that sensation in your jaw. For many people, this can be accomplished in a minute or two.

- To convince yourself that you can control your pain, use hypnosis and concentrate on making a part of your body itch. Focus on the sensation of itching, and make it appear somewhere on your body, perhaps on your hand or foot. When you feel the itch and when it demands scratching, switch to another technique involving active fantasy. See yourself in a pleasant situation of your choosing. You will notice that you have "forgotten" the itch (you gain more control). You didn't have to scratch the itch you created, you forgot it (turned it off) (Yates & Wallace, 1984).

One helpful and fairly simple method to help you fall asleep, particularly if your pain is keeping you awake, is what I call "programming." Imagine placing a kitchen timer in your head. You may be able to actually see it in your mind — white with black numbers, one through ten, and a pointer like a hand on a clock. Starting with one, the pointer slowly ticks past each number. As it gets closer and closer to ten, you become sleepier and sleepier, and when it reaches number ten, you just might fall asleep. It almost sounds too simple, but the mind is really very powerful.

EMG (Electromyographic) Biofeedback

Biofeedback is a technique that teaches patients to recognize and control bodily functions previously thought to be involuntary, such as breathing, heart rate, blood pressure, skin temperature, brain wave patterns, muscle tension, and sweat gland activity. It is based on the theory that the mind controls the body and, therefore, most — if not all — physiological functions can be brought under voluntary control.

Biofeedback is painless and non-invasive. Proponents believe it can be used to alleviate chronic pain, stress, and physical symptoms associated with TMJ, back and neck pain, migraine, muscle spasm, tinnitus, hypertension, insomnia, peptic ulcers, epilepsy, diabetes, and even drug and alcohol addictions.

For the TMJ sufferer, EMG is used to measure variations in muscle activity. Electrodes are attached to a particular muscle, usually starting with the masseter and progressing through the neck, shoulder, and back muscles. The patient is instructed to concentrate on the muscle and to visualize it as being relaxed. If the muscle contracts even slightly, faint electrical impulses are detected by the electrodes, sent to a machine, amplified, and transformed into either visual or auditory output, such as flashing lights or a beeping sound. The stronger and longer the muscle contraction, the stronger the output. In effect, the machine feeds back information regarding muscle activity, a physiological process. By observing the output, the patient learns to relax and control the degree of muscle spasm. Many patients are able to significantly decrease bruxism with just 20 minutes of practice.

Training generally consists of several supervised sessions, followed by home practice using a portable monitor. The ultimate goal is for the patient to wean himself off the machine completely. In most cases, some pain relief is seen after four to six weeks, although training usually continues for about six months with sessions gradually tapering off. Often, various forms of relaxation, such as progressive muscle relaxation and autogenic tapes, are used in conjunction with biofeedback.

It is claimed that many TMJ sufferers are able to lessen their dependency on medication, or even discontinue it entirely, with the help of biofeedback. In order to be successful, however, you must be motivated and willing to practice regularly and complete all the sessions. According to the ADA, EMG biofeedback "has reasonable scientific support" (ADA, 1989).

Humor and Laughter

Laughter is very healthy, just as crying is sometimes. It increases your heart rate, releases endorphins, reduces stress, and stimulates your immune system.

If you can laugh at your situation, it is much easier to put it in perspective. A good friend of mine who has had numerous surgeries and I sometimes break into hysterical giggles when we are having lunch together, cutting our cheeseburgers into tiny bites with a knife and fork. And my children can't help but laugh when a pea drops out of my mouth during dinner. Sometimes when we are out eating at the mall, my husband orders a huge submarine with steak and all the fixins'. He can't resist holding it next to my mouth, saying, "Do you think you can take a bite out of this?"

Many times my husband and I, while waiting in yet another examination room for "one more opinion," imagine the doctor sitting in his office, rubbing his hands together with greed, hoping that his next patient will be riddled with TMJ problems severe enough to warrant a $5,000 operation so that he can take a trip to the Bahamas. Other times we visualize the orthodontist I used to go to, in his office with the door shut and shades drawn, doctoring x-rays so it looks as though his newest patient has a really serious problem — one that will require several thousand dollars worth of braces. After all, his wife has been nagging and nagging about that brand new car. A sense of humor really does go a long way towards helping us to cope and survive.

Chapter 15

Going to the Doctor

"It's not enough for doctors to stop playing God. The rest of us must get up off our knees."
Editor, Medical Self-Care magazine

People in pain are anxious to believe that their doctors know what they are doing and are going to make them better. After all, isn't that what doctors are for? In the field of TMJ where so much controversy exists, it is easy to fall victim to unscrupulous doctors who are more concerned with how much money they can get from you than making you better.

Quackery

Quackery has been defined as "the promotion of false or unproven methods for profit, usually without the patient's informed consent." Dr. John Dodes, DDS, says, "Quackery is easy and lucrative. The only skill it requires is the ability to look a patient in the eye, lie to him, and take his money" (Remba, 1987).

It's hard to believe, but in the *ADA News* (April 6, 1981) there was an advertisement for the "only TMJ seminar that will show you how to tap unused dental and medical insurance resources and build on your already-existing practice." It was entitled, "How to Increase, Revitalize, and Inflation-Proof Your Practice Through TMJ." Such ads are attractive to business-oriented dentists who may or may not believe in the treatments such seminars are pushing.

According to Enid Neidle, ADA's former director of scientific affairs, dental education is partly to blame. "Where dental schools have done an exceedingly poor job, and continue to do so, is to incorporate those things into the curriculum that will create in their graduates an inquiring mind, a respect for science, a comprehension of what research means, and a deep understanding of how fundamental to the practice of dentistry scientifically generated knowledge is" (Neidle, 1990).

The scientific method, scientific reasoning, and statistics are not emphasized in dental education and, as a result, many students are willing to accept the views of a perceived authority figure without demanding to know the science supporting those views. Instructors teach what they happen to believe and, too often, their information is either unproven or disproven. Many prestigious dental schools or reputable professional groups sponsor courses eligible for official continuing education credit. It is easy to mistakenly conclude that the courses are scientifically valid (Dodes, April 1991).

In order for a treatment to be considered scientific, it must be proven to work through rigorous scientific testing. "Anecdotes, testimonials, untested observations, and personal beliefs do not meet the criteria for determining the value and validity of a treatment" (Berry, 1987).

You are probably asking yourself, "Isn't quackery against the law?" Actually anti-quackery laws *do* exist, but prosecution expenses are astronomical, so the FDA generally does not take action against "economic fraud" products or services which are worthless, but not dangerous. Another problem is that it's "very difficult to get a patient to testify against a quack. Patients believe the quack is giving them a cure that's on the cutting edge of science" (Remba, 1987).

What You Must Know Before Going to the Doctor

One of the most common requests The TMJ Association receives is for a doctor referral. Considering the iatrogenic aspect of TMJ disorders, we cannot offer physician referrals. But we can help you avoid dangerous medical pitfalls.

- Professionals in the field of TMJ don't agree on much of anything. Doctors differ drastically as to how problems should be treated and what really constitutes a problem. You have, no doubt, already run into many medical professionals who have many different opinions and attitudes about TMJ. Since most doctors are excellent salesmen, often it is difficult to know which ones can be trusted and which ones should be avoided.

- There is no required certification to treat TMJ disorders. Too many patients are impressed with so-called "specialists" whose "credentials" often amount to nothing more than a piece of paper obtained by attending a weekend seminar sponsored by a "TMJ organization" that is unrecognized and unscientific (Dodes, Oct. 1991).

- With no standards of care, many doctors are experimenting with new procedures that don't have much of a track record and certainly cannot have an adequate period of follow up. Many current treatments have never been proven to be safe or effective, and in some cases, do more harm than good.

- Throughout your search for relief, always keep in mind that TMJ is big business, and a lot of doctors are getting in on the act and making a lot of money in the process.

- Remember that most people with TMJ symptoms don't need medical treatment. Chances are excellent that you will get better with simple, expensive treatments you can do yourself at home. If you really feel you need medical help, there are a couple of things you should do.

Educate yourself.

Find out as much as you can by reading and talking to other sufferers. There is nothing more valuable than talking to someone who has been there and learning from his or her experience. An informed patient knows how to talk to a doctor and what questions to ask. Learn all the facts about your condition and explore all options.

Proceed with caution.

Take your time and proceed very carefully. It may mean the difference in receiving satisfactory treatment and eventually becoming pain free, and the heartache of spending the rest of your life wishing things had been done differently. For those of you who are considering any kind of TMJ treatment, either conservative or radical, you must never forget that once your body has been damaged, it may be too late to turn back.

Finding a Doctor

When you talk to other sufferers, find out what doctors they have seen and how they felt about them and the treatment they received. If you have a family doctor you trust, ask him to recommend someone who is experienced with the conservative treatment of TMJ problems.

Some experts suggest starting with a dentist, oral surgeon, or orthodontist, while others may say a psychiatrist, chiropractor, or physical therapist is the place to begin. The problem you may run into is that the doctor you choose will more than likely suggest treatment that he is qualified to provide. In other words, if you see an orthodontist first, he may very well decide that you need dental appliances and/or braces, whereas an oral surgeon may insist that your condition warrants a surgical procedure.

Even a dentist may want to start out with a splint, or appliance, and many dentists are actually doing orthodontics now as well. If you choose a doctor who is not familiar with TMJ disorders, he may eventually refer you to a psychologist or psychiatrist, insisting you are a hypochondriac, implying that you enjoy your pain. Or he may experiment with a variety of drugs until one is found that relieves your symptoms. The problem here is that your symptoms are being covered up and not actually treated. In such cases, addiction is a very real danger as is the agony of withdrawal.

Making an appointment

If possible, choose an appointment time when you think you will be the most rested and in the least amount of pain. A late morning appointment might be best; you don't have to be up at the crack of dawn, but, on the other hand, you won't be tired before you even get to the doctor's office. When you call to schedule an appointment, be sure to tell the receptionist that you want ample time — it's not unusual to need one, two, or even three hours for a consultation.

Before you go

Arrange for your spouse, family member, or a close friend to go with you to help you listen and ask questions. Sometimes it is difficult to be objective about yourself; someone who knows you may be able to provide the doctor with important information. Often, patients begin to think their pain, and the many changes that have been inflicted on their lives as a result, are normal. A friend or family member remembers you the way you used to be.

Make a detailed list of your symptoms. Note when they first started, what seems to make them worse, what helps (if anything), their intensity and frequency, and the time of day when they are the worst. Think about your overall health and to what extent your pain and other symptoms affect you on a daily basis — your family, your job, and your social life.

Write down all of your questions and concerns. Don't leave anything out because you are afraid of sounding stupid. No question is stupid. And something you may think is meaningless may be important to the doctor.

Write Down Your History, Don't try to recreate your medical history off the top of your head; it can be difficult and exhausting. Also, when you go to the doctor, you may be nervous or frightened and it is easy to forget something, especially if you're in a lot of pain. (If you are handed a 10-page questionnaire in the doctor's office, having a written history will make your job a lot easier.) This is very important, so take your time and be as accurate and thorough as possible. (Ask someone to help you remember everything.)

Be sure to include the following information: any previous treatment such as orthodontics, equilibration, extractions, appliances, steroid injections, and surgery (note dates, doctors, and results); any medications (dosage, frequency, how long you've been taking them, and allergies and sensitivities, if any); accidents such as a whiplash or head injury; and any other medical conditions the doctor should know about.

Then gather together all your x-rays, x-ray reports, models, appliances, before and after photos of yourself, OP reports, notes of previous consultations — anything you have. Be sure to make copies of all written documentation, including your own history. If another doctor has any of your records, allow plenty of time to get them. (To obtain copies of your medical records, all you need to do is ask, usually in writing. However, laws vary from state to state, so it's a good idea to check.) Once you have assembled your records, put everything in a large box and keep them together for future consultations.

At the Doctor's Office

After filling out insurance forms, you will probably see the doctor in a consultation room. He will start by asking you a lot of questions. This is your chance to give him a copy of your history, and then he will examine you. This may include range of motion tests, listening to your jaw joints with a stethoscope, and palpation of your jaw, neck, shoulders, and head. He may also take a few x-rays. When the examination is finished, there are some important questions you should ask. It is a really good idea to take notes or, better yet, have the person who goes with you take notes; you will not remember everything after you leave. If you do not understand something, say so. Ask your doctor:

- What is wrong with me?
- What is causing the problem?
- Is there anything I can do to help myself?
- What do you recommend?
- How much will the treatment cost?
- How long will the treatment take?
- What are the chances for success? A complete recovery or significant improvement?
- What alternatives do I have?
- Will you be working with any other doctors on my case? (A team approach can be important.)

An Important Word About TMJ Treatments

There are several dozen treatment modalities for TMJ disorders. As you seek help, you must keep in mind that most of them have never been scientifically proven to be safe or effective for TMJ.

"The key words to keep in mind about TMJ treatment are 'conservative' and 'reversible.' Conservative treatments are as simple as possible and do not invade the tissues of the face, jaw, or joint." These include moist heat, ice, a soft diet, over-the-counter analgesics (pain killers), and relaxation techniques. "Reversible treatments do not cause permanent, or irreversible, changes in the structure or position of the jaw or teeth," and are aimed at relieving pain and muscle spasm and improving joint function, just as treatments for other joints in the body (NIDR, 1993).

Before you leave

Ask the doctor to recommend at least one doctor for another opinion. Request copies of any x-rays he has taken as well as test results. Ask for a letter to send to your insurance company that explains your condition as well as the treatment required and why.

IMPORTANT: If a doctor tells you that you need surgery, remember, very few TMJ sufferers even *need* surgery. Surgery is fraught with countless risks and, in many cases, hurts more than it helps.

If your doctor insists surgery is the only answer for you, ask him:

- Is there a physical problem within the joints — not just muscle spasm?
- What are the risks? There is always a risk with general anesthesia, and there are plenty of risks with TMJ surgery — some extremely serious — especially with any type of implant.
- What can I expect in the way of results?

- Has everything else been tried?
- What if I don't have surgery?
- How much surgery have you done? A doctor should do surgery regularly enough to be experienced and stay in practice but not so much that he is conducting an all-day assembly line in the operating room.
- What about post-op physical therapy? If you don't have it, you may very well end up worse in the long run.

It's a good idea to ask for the names of several patients who have had surgery and talk to them. If the doctor is hesitant to give you names or only offers you one or two, you should wonder why he doesn't want you talking to his patients. (Often doctors don't follow up their patients longer than a few months. You want to know how they are doing a year, two years, even five years later.)

In addition, ask yourself:

- Have other doctors (besides surgeons) agreed that I need surgery?
- Is my pain physically and emotionally debilitating? Is it so bad that I can no longer go on the way I am?
- Am I willing to have surgery knowing that there is no guarantee and that it could actually make me worse? Once you have surgery, you may be in for a lifetime of more surgery — a miserable and never-ending alternative.

Doctor "Shoulds" and "Should Nots"

Your doctor should:

- treat you like a human being. This should go without saying, but a doctor who treats you with respect may be hard to find. You should trust the doctor and feel that he is genuinely concerned about you.

- listen to you and answer all of your questions thoroughly and to your satisfaction.

- allow you plenty of time.

- try conservative treatments first.

- encourage you to seek other opinions and offer you referrals.

- give you names of his patients you can talk with. Usually patients don't tell their doctors everything; they will be more honest and open with another TMJ sufferer.

- be willing to work with other doctors towards a pre-established goal — not just flounder around from one treatment to another.

Your doctor should not:

- hurry you or avoid your questions.

- order unnecessary x-rays, particularly if you have already had dozens and you have some recent ones with you.

- jump to the conclusion that you have a TMJ disorder because your joints pop or click. Most experts agree that, without other symptoms, a clicking or popping joint is nothing to worry about.

- rush into irreversible and/or expensive treatments including repositioning splint therapy, steroid injections, orthodontics, equilibration, or surgery. (He should also be careful about recommending long-term use of drugs such as painkillers, tranquilizers, or antidepressants.)

- tell you that you know too much, you read too much, you're seeing too many doctors, your pain is all in your head, or you enjoy your pain. If he does, find another doctor.

- "Stop seeing your doctor as God and do not be overwhelmed by his personality and bedside manner." This advice comes from John Dodes, DDS of Woodhaven, NY. He goes on to say, "There is scientific information available to doctors which indicates that invasive procedures are not working and, are in fact, making patients worse. Many doctors do not want to accept this consensus because it is not financially rewarding" (Dodes, Oct. 1991).

I personally would stay away from a doctor who is a member of a TMJ organization or president of a foundation he established himself — his intentions may not be completely unbiased or even honest. Any professional who devotes his entire practice to the treatment of TMJ disorders may only be interested in making money by telling everyone who comes into his office that he or she has a TMJ problem. Be wary of any doctor who says he is the only one who can cure you.

If you have already had surgery and other irreversible treatments, you must stop being your doctor's subject and start being an advocate for yourself. Become an active participant in your treatment. Perhaps you can at least keep yourself from getting any worse.

A final word: If you suspect that you have been a victim of dental quackery, contact your local dental society and your state attorney general. You can also contact the Victim Redress Committee of the National Council Against Health Fraud, c/o Stephen Barrett, M.D., P.O. Box 1747, Allentown, PA 18105.

General Reminders:
- Be educated.
- Do what you can to help yourself.
- Get as many opinions as you want or need to be satisfied.

- See several different kinds of doctors. A surgeon does surgery — that's how he makes his living. An orthodontist does braces. Each doctor treats what he has been trained to treat. (I would personally be leery of a doctor who treats TMJ and nothing else; he may not *see* anything else.)

- Doctors are not perfect. There is admittedly a lot of quackery going on and even honest doctors with good intentions make mistakes. A doctor should not be afraid to say, "I don't know." If he can't answer a question, he should say so and either try to find out or send you to a doctor who can.

- The field of TMJ is very controversial. Doctors don't agree on much — if anything. New treatments are continually being developed and a lot of experimentation is going on. Most treatments have never been proven to be safe and effective and may do more harm than good.

- Most TMJ problems are actually Myofascial Pain Dysfunction (MPD) and can be treated with safe, conservative methods or no treatment at all.

- Most patients do not need surgery! If a doctor recommends surgery before trying anything else, I would find another doctor.

- Take your time and don't rush into any treatment; you may spend the rest of your life wishing things had been done differently.

- TMJ is not cheap! You can spend thousands of dollars in your search for relief and some insurance companies won't touch it.

- It's your body, your time, and your money!

Chapter 16

The Insurance Dilemma

Julie had 19 surgeries and still lives a life of excruciating pain. Sometimes it is so severe that she is screaming, even after 200 milligrams of morphine. Every day of her life is a struggle against suicide.

When you are in pain, worrying about paying your medical bills should be the last thing on your mind. TMJ sufferers already have more than enough stress in their lives. Unfortunately, many insurance companies provide little, if any coverage for the treatment of TMJ disorders. For many sufferers and their families, the financial burden becomes yet another chapter in a seemingly never-ending nightmare.

One of the most frustrating problems faced by people with TMJ is trying to obtain insurance coverage. Many medical and dental insurance plans do not provide coverage for the treatment of jaw joint disorders. Some offer very limited coverage, perhaps on an individual, case-by-case basis, or with strict stipulations. For example, an evaluation may be covered but not treatment. Or some companies have either annual or lifetime fee limits even though they wouldn't dream of setting limits on treatment for a knee condition or problems in other joints in the body. Still others will pay for surgery but refuse to cover conservative therapies.

The policy regarding treatment of TMJ disorders can vary widely from one insurance company to another. Some companies want proof (for example, an x-ray) of an internal problem such as bone degeneration or a damaged disc, and may be willing to pay for surgery. This is unfortunate since muscle spasm, although not visible on an x-ray, can cause excruciating and often disabling pain.

If your insurance company views TMJ as a dental condition and you do not have dental coverage, then they may not be willing to pay your TMJ expenses. It may depend on what kind of doctor you consult for your condition. If you begin with a medical doctor such as an orthopedist or ENT, for example, your insurance company might provide coverage for their treatment claims simply because they are coming from an MD. But if you start with an orthodontist, dentist, or oral surgeon, the insurance company may automatically think "dental" and refuse any coverage on that basis. A company may be willing to pay for treatment performed by someone other than a dentist or orthodontist. That's because there is so much controversy about whether TMJ is a medical or dental problem.

For the majority of TMJ sufferers, a medical team approach is needed and can end up costing a small fortune. Without insurance coverage, many people may go without treatment altogether. Some experts fear this neglect simply allows minor TMJ problems to develop into serious ones that may eventually require surgery.

On the other hand, one can't help but wonder if such people might actually be far better off using self-help treatments at home and avoiding professional medical intervention. Perhaps those of us whose insurance companies won't cover our TMJ medical bills are really the lucky ones. Who can say?

The people most affected by a lack of coverage are implant victims who are in desperate need of implant removal, follow-up care, multiple future revision surgeries — which can cost between $35,000 and $85,000 — and drug maintenance for chronic and often debilitating pain they will face for the rest of their lives as the result of their failed implants. Ironically, some companies who wouldn't cover conservative therapies and yet paid for surgery and, in some cases the implantation of various types of untested devices to replace all or part of the jaw joint, have refused to pay to have failed implants removed, saying this is "experimental."

The problem with TMJ and insurance coverage is a complex one with several major points that need to be addressed:

1. Are TMJ disorders medical or dental? Both professions are treating them. Although the close relationship between the jaw joints and the teeth cannot be ignored, and one directly affects the other, the TMJ is a joint much like all the others in the body, just more complex. To further add to the confusion, symptoms may appear in many different parts of the body.

2. Who is qualified to treat TMJ disorders? It has been said that TMJ is not a mandatory course in the dental school curriculum. There is no specialty certification required to treat TMJ problems. Almost every kind of doctor around is "jumping on the TMJ treatment bandwagon."

3. How should TMJ disorders be treated? According to one source, more than fifty treatment modalities currently exist. There is no conclusive scientific research to tell which ones are effective and which ones are not. With no standards of care, doctors are trying just about everything and a lot of experimentation is going on.

4. Current treatment costs are astronomical. By the time a

patient gets bounced back and forth among half a dozen "specialists," the medical bills can easily add up to thousands of dollars. Where does it end?

With no medical or dental specialty certification required to treat TMJ, and no consensus on definition or standards of care at this point, insurance companies claim to be protecting themselves from exorbitant costs. And, until the situation changes, many insurance companies may continue to enforce strict guidelines and refuse coverage for TMJ care. In the meantime, one expert has the following advice for doctors:

- Submit TMJ claims under major medical instead of dental.
- Provide the insurance company with a brief report of the patient's case.
- Indicate diagnosis with terms such as "degenerative arthritis" (avoid vague terms such as "TMJ syndrome").
- Settle with an arbitrator if a claim is denied (Lader & Vander, 1987).

Dr. Henry Dutson, orthodontist in Annandale, VA, advises doctors to document ways in which the symptoms of the disorder medically inhibit the sufferer. For instance, the inability to eat properly and obtain adequate nutrition may be causing weight loss or other health problems. The idea is to provide the insurance company with information that will convince them that treatment is a medical necessity.

It may also be helpful if **medical** doctors write letters to the insurance company to back up what the dentist is saying (Dutson, Oct. 1991). Some insurance representatives cringe at any TMJ claims that come across their desks, particularly if they are from a dentist or orthodontist.

You may be asking, is there anything the patient can do? The answer is a most definite yes! Write letters explaining the degree to which your life is affected, for example, your inability to function as a wife and mother, hold down your job, or obtain adequate nutrition. Call and ask to speak to a claim representative and explain your situation. It may help to make a bit of a nuisance of yourself. Part of the trouble is that many patients do not know what coverage they have and may automatically assume their insurance will not pay for TMJ treatment. Some won't question their insurance companies and possibly don't appeal in the event their claims are denied. Often, if patients make enough noise long enough and loud enough, they will be successful. As Henry Dutson says, "Out of every 10 people, one of them will fight; the other 9 accept the rules the way they are. The one person who fights usually wins" (Dutson, Oct. 1991).

In recent years, several states have taken steps to mandate at least some degree of coverage for TMJ disorders:

Arkansas: TMJ disorders must be treated the same as any other illness or injury and not considered dental work.

Georgia: Claims for treatment by a physician or a dentist for orofacial pain including, but not limited to, TMJ and myofascial pain problems must be honored under major medical policies of insurers and not-for-profit service corporations.

Kentucky: All policies and contracts that provide coverage for surgical or non-surgical treatment of skeletal disorders must provide coverage for medically necessary procedures relating to TMJ and craniomandibular disorders.

Maryland: Group and individual insurers and non-profit health-service plans that provide coverage for diagnostic or surgical procedures involving a bone or a joint of the skeletal structure must provide coverage for the same procedure involving a bone or joint of the face, neck, or head if medically necessary to treat a congenital deformity, disease, or injury.

Minnesota: Insurers, HMOs, and subscriber contracts must provide coverage for treatment of TMJ disorders when administered by doctors or dentists.

Nevada: Legislation prohibits insurance policies and contracts from excluding, either by specific language or settlement practices, coverage of the temporomandibular joint. Methods of treatment that are recognized as dental procedures, however, may be excluded, and insurers may limit TMJ benefits to 50 percent of usual charges and to treatment that is medically necessary. [Who decides what is medically necessary?]

New Mexico: All insurers must provide coverage for surgical and non-surgical treatment of TMJ and craniomandibular disorders, subject to the same conditions, limitations, prior review, and referral procedures that are applicable to treatment of any other body joint.

North Dakota: Coverage for TMJ disorders must be provided in all but special disease policies. Coverage applies if treatment is administered or prescribed by a physician, dentist, or surgeon. Benefits may be limited to a lifetime maximum of $8,000 per person for surgery and $2,000 for non-surgical treatment. [In light of current costs, this could be spent real quick!]

Tennessee: Accident and health policies must cover treatment of TMJ disorders by a dentist when such treatment also could be performed by a physician.

Texas: Orthodontic coverage may not be excluded on grounds that overbite, overjet, openbite, or arch length discrepancies measure less than 4 millimeters. Also, HMOs must provide treatment for the temporomandibular and craniomandibular joints when comparable to diagnostic and/or surgical treatment of skeletal joints in other parts of the body.

Vermont: Treatment of TMJ disorders does not come within standard dental care and treatment exclusion and must be honored under the medical expense portion of the policy.

Washington: Surgical and non-surgical TMJ benefits must

be offered as optional coverage in medical and dental group insurance contracts.

West Virginia: Insurers must make coverage available for TMJ and craniomandibular disorders pursuant to standards developed by the insurance commissioner (Zaejian, 1991).

To find out what the policy is regarding TMJ coverage in your state, contact your state insurance commissioner.

Legislation pending in some states attempts to prevent insurance companies from discriminating against diagnosis and treatment of bones and joints of the head and neck. In other words, if a particular diagnostic or treatment procedure is covered when performed on the knee, for example, that same procedure could not be denied or excluded solely because the procedure is performed on the TMJ.

One of the main goals of The TMJ Association is to stimulate further discussion of the insurance dilemma with various congressional committees.

Chapter 17

Coping Strategies
for You and Your Family

Sally says she feels useless. Her life has been torn away from her and she can no longer do the things she used to do and enjoy. At twenty-one, she managed a restaurant and was a part-time model. Now her face is mutilated from operation after operation and she spends most of her time in bed eating ice cream and crying.

For many TMJ sufferers, pain is a way of life. It is present every minute of every day. Chronic pain of any kind is exhausting. It depletes your body of the strength and energy needed to carry out the routines of day-to-day living. It interferes with, and eventually begins to take over, the lives of the sufferer and the family — with devastating effects. Many TMJ patients become desperate enough to try anything. Most patients believe what their doctors tell them and may submit to harmful, unproven treatments that may make them worse.

Unfortunately, doctors are not taught how to diagnose and treat pain in medical school. For this reason, pain is frequently mismanaged or ignored. Because they are inadequately educated about pain and can't find proof of its existence beyond the patient's description, doctors often dismiss their complaints as imaginary or exaggerated.

Many TMJ patients have gone from doctor to doctor and no one has diagnosed their problem. The patient, as well as friends and family, may very well agree with the doctor that the pain is imagined. After all, many TMJ sufferers look fine. Their pain is not so obvious. And it doesn't show up on an x-ray like a fracture, for example.

Depression

It is no wonder that many patients become depressed. Depression is probably one of the most common and difficult problems TMJ sufferers face. When you are in pain, your quality of life is diminished. Often you cannot do the things you used to do, and this is extremely hard for some people to accept.

Part of chronic pain is the grief process. A patient whose life has been changed drastically feels a tremendous sense of loss. They may feel that their problems are never going to go away, that they will never go back to the way they used to be, or have what they had at one time. Some feel as though they are different, that they will never be the same spouse or parent they once were. And for many this is true. They can't go back. Those good times are gone and there's a loss because of it and it makes them sad. It doesn't help to deny the truth. It is better to admit it, but it doesn't help to dwell on it for long. The first step towards feeling better is understanding the truth of what has happened and taking steps to deal with it.

Important: If you are depressed to the point of suicide, you need to get help. If money's a problem, call a suicide prevention hotline for referrals to affordable counseling. Help is out there for those who need it. You are not alone.

Sex and Chronic Pain

Approximately 75% of chronic pain sufferers experience some degree of sexual dysfunction. People with chronic pain are often exhausted and depressed, and fear that sex will increase their pain. This seems to be especially true for TMJ sufferers. For many, even kissing can be very painful.

Unfortunately, many patients are hesitant to discuss their problems and the situation is not resolved. This adds even more stress. Often, doctors don't address problems related to sex, perhaps because they are not experienced in doing so or they are embarrassed. But sexual concerns are a legitimate concern that merits recognition and resolution. Some of the following suggestions may help you if you are having problems with intimacy.

- If something you do sexually increases your pain, stop doing it and try something else. If one position for intercourse, for example, causes pain, try another position. Sexual response, which may be deadened by chronic pain, can come from simply touching. Try different things until you find one that is pleasurable for you. Remember that all people need to be loved, caressed, and held.

- Physical intimacy can actually increase our ability to manage pain. Sex promotes relaxation and increases the body's production of endorphins which are natural painkillers.

- Some people find they have more successful sex lives if they learn techniques that lessen their pain and help them relax, such as self-hypnosis, visualization, or even listening to music they enjoy.

- It is important to pace yourself throughout the day so you have some energy for sex. You may have to schedule time for sex just as you do for other activities.

- Do what you can to improve your desire, experimenting a little if necessary. If you are both patient, you may be able to attain some degree of sexual fulfillment. Tell your partner what hurts and what doesn't. Often the healthy partner is afraid to initiate sex because he might hurt you or feel rejected if you don't respond. One patient says herhusband no longer approachs her; he waits for her wives to make the first move. That way, he knows that her pain is at least under control enough that she can be close without causing more pain. Whenever possible, reach out to your spouse first.

- Communicate openly with your partner. Sometimes just talking about this problem can go a long way toward solving it. It's at least a first step in the right direction (Gendleman, 1989).

Reasons and Ways to Survive and Go On

I'll never forget the phone conversation I had with Janet one night. Right in the middle of a sentence, she sobbed and said, "Oh my God, the pain is so bad, I just wish somebody was here to hold me." I felt as though my heart was being wrenched out of my chest. Fighting back my own tears, I said to her, "I'm so sorry. If only there was something I could to do help you." Then she told me I had already helped her more than I would ever know, just by listening and sharing her pain over the telephone.

How do you convince a patient who has had so many surgeries she's lost count, is still in agony, her doctors have given her up for crazy, she's just existing in a life of unbearable pain ... how do you convince her that life is worth living? Many

TMJ sufferers are in so much pain, so non-functional, so depressed, and their lives are so totally devastated, that it is difficult — if not impossible — to know what to say to offer them comfort or hope.

Many feel they have no meaning in their lives anymore. They are just hanging on. They do not deserve what has happened to them. They are victims who have been terribly wronged by their doctors. But how do they move beyond the tragedy of their lives? How do they see that there is still good to be found? Something to live for?

What I really hate to hear, so I'm sure most other people do too, is "Cheer up, it could be a lot worse. You could have cancer or AIDS." It's kind of like telling a paraplegic that he could be a quadriplegic and have no use of his arms *or* legs. But there is some truth here. Sometimes it helps to put your situation into its proper perspective and, even if it does sound a bit cold, to tell yourself you really could be a lot worse.

Ann has a unique way of dealing with her pain. When she's having a bad day, she recalls the worst day she can remember and compares the pain she's presently experiencing with the most excruciating she's ever had. This probably won't work for everybody, but it might help some of you. I can't help but marvel at the many ways TMJ sufferers find to cope with their pain and all the problems that come along with it. We are really very resourceful human beings because we have to be.

For most of you, no matter what stage your TMJ disorder is in, there is something — no matter how small — that may be enough to keep you fighting through another day. Try some of these coping techniques:

- Don't look past getting through today — the next minute, the next hour. Take small steps. Think of your pain in 24-hour cycles that you can manage. Try setting small attainable goals each day and do whatever it takes to accomplish them. On a bad day, one goal may be as simple as getting out of bed and dressing. That's okay. The important thing is you have accomplished whatever it is you set out to do. Be proud of yourself. It helps to keep a positive attitude and think about progress in terms of inches and not great strides. We all need successes, even small ones.

- Every day choose something — even one thing — that you like to do and do it. Remember that little things count and can improve the way you feel. Even if it's just a nice long soak in a warm tub or a picnic in the back yard with your kids, the important thing is that you've let yourself enjoy something, even for a short while. Watch something you enjoy on TV. Listen to some classical music — it can be very soothing. Read. Books are one of the greatest escapes. When you are lost in a book, it is hard to feel sorry for yourself or even think about your own problems. Do whatever makes you feel like a human being.

- Set a reasonable schedule and try to stick with it. Set your alarm for the same time each morning and when it rings, get out of bed. Of course, allow yourself extra rest and naps when you need them. On bad days, pamper yourself. You deserve it.

- Try not to spend the day in bed with the shades drawn. If at all possible, get up, get dressed, and tell yourself there's a good chance you will feel better as the day goes on. You just might be in for a pleasant surprise. As Becky has found, even on her worst days, by the time she showers, puts on her best suit, fixes her face and hair, and gets in the car to run errands, she "almost feels human." And she's always surprised. She feels very strongly that it's important to hold onto your vanity. It means you care about who you are and how you look to other people. Even if you don't feel this is important, if you try it for a while, you may soon begin to feel better.

- Make an effort to get outside whenever you possibly can and look at the world around you. Try taking a short walk in the rain, plant some flowers, or buy a bird feeder and watch the many different kinds of birds that will visit your yard. Do what you can to be a part of life. If you really can't, sit by an open window. Inhale deeply, breathing in the fresh air and sunshine.

- Write down your feelings. Sometimes just facing our fears and problems is the first step towards finding ways to make life a little more bearable.

- Allow yourself to cry. It can be a tremendous release and, not only that, it's healthy.

- Remember that you have no reason to feel ashamed or guilty. Amy cooks and cleans her house almost compulsively, when she has no right being out of bed. But she does it because, as she says, "It's the only thing I can do and feel good about." She feels as though she's no good to anyone as a human being, but she can deal with the housework and feel a sense of accomplishment. If she could only realize that there are people who care about her and that she has a lot to offer. All of us have something to offer other human beings — the wisdom gained from our own experience, a little bit of strength, a small piece of hope, our love. Other people need you and care about you.

- Know that it is okay to feel anger. What has happened to some patients I have spoken with shouldn't have happened to a dog. Scream. Yell. Throw something (please choose something that won't break). Anger can be productive because it encourages us to take control and do something to change things we are not happy with. It is partly anger that prompted me to write this book — anger and outrage at the lives so many TMJ sufferers are living.

- Do something for someone else. You may forget your own problems for a short time. You will dwell less on yourself if you are involved with helping others. And you'll feel good about yourself and less isolated. Maria's father recently had a heart attack and she had to go out of town to be with her mother through a very difficult time. When she left, she was in absolute agony, to the point of being bedridden, but when she returned, she found that she had forgotten all about her pain. Perhaps it would have improved anyway, but it's possible that she became so involved in her concern for her family that she was able to put her own suffering aside.

- Surround yourself with people who will make you feel better, physically and emotionally. Susan's parents have had a hard time accepting her condition and the restrictions it has placed on her life. Her mother says things like, "If you'd just get up out of that bed and get dressed and stop feeling so sorry for yourself and being so selfish, you'd be okay." It's not that she doesn't care about her daughter or even that she is being cruel. I think that she simply cannot stand to watch Susan suffer and she doesn't know how to handle it.

  Hopefully, when she can accept the situation, she will be a stronger source of support for her daughter. I'm not saying you need someone who will pity you and wait on you hand and foot, but you do need people who understand and acknowledge how you feel and try to make you feel better. Sometimes it's enough for someone to validate your pain, to tell you they understand and know how you feel.

- Be with children whenever possible. They have an amazing way of making us smile when we are at our lowest. Even if you are having a really bad day and can't get out of bed, you can snuggle under the covers and read or just talk. Children need adults to listen to them and hug and kiss them. You can do this. You will be surprised at how understanding and attentive they can be.

- Be honest with family and friends about your feelings. Don't expect them to know what you are going through if you don't show them in some way. Believe me, people do care. Don't shut them out; give them a chance. When you are really feeling bad, don't try to do too much. Ask for help. You may be surprised at people's reactions.

- Don't be afraid to ask for emotional support from family and friends. Sometimes all you need is for someone to listen or a shoulder to cry on. If necessary, ask for a hug when you need it the most.

- On your worst days, try to arrange for someone — a family member or good friend — to be with you. It is a lot easier to see the bright side of life (yes, there is one) and cope when you are not alone.

- Focus on what you can do, not what you can no longer do. We have all heard the Serenity Prayer used by Alcoholics Anonymous. "God, grant me the serenity to accept the things I cannot change, the courage to change the things I can, and the wisdom to know the difference."

- Try praying. This is difficult, I know, because after living through years of absolute hell, if you are like many sufferers, you start to wonder where God is through all your pain and suffering. Once when I was talking with Melanie on the phone, she told me that she didn't know how much longer she could go on. I asked her if there was anything I could do to help and she said, "Pray for me. Maybe God will listen to someone else. I don't pray for myself anymore, I just ask Him to take care of my children." When I got off the phone, I discovered that, in a way, prayer is a lot like meditation. Perhaps it was just "thinking out loud" about Melanie and her anguish, but I knew God was listening. Sometimes prayer is all we have left.

With TMJ, everyone — not just the patient — becomes a victim. However, it is vital that it does not become the primary focus of everyone's lives. TMJ cannot be allowed to take over the entire family. Here are some suggestions that will hopefully make things run a little more smoothly for you and your family.

- Take the time to tell your family they are important to you and you love them. Hug your kids. Kiss your spouse. The human touch is vital for existence. Reach out to others.

- Whenever you can, do things with your family and/or friends. Participate in games and outings. If you don't feel up to it, encourage them to go on without you, casually but firmly assuring them that you will be just fine.

- Allow your family to be human. No one can be wonderful, perfect, and supportive 100% of the time. Let them show their emotions. Remember, it's painful for them to watch you suffer and worry about what's going to happen next. Sometimes the TMJ sufferer needs to comfort the healthy spouse.

- Encourage your spouse and children to get away occasionally. It's important for them to take a breather sometimes. They will return more supportive and refreshed.

- Don't complain when you don't have to. Your family often knows how you feel. Try not to make this the focal point of your family. It's not fair to your husband and your children and it's not fair to you. You deserve better and so do they.

  Debbie's husband goes to the gym several times a week to work out. Since she thinks it is very important that they do things together whenever possible, she occasionally goes along. The last time, as usual, she overdid it and worked out a little bit too hard. As she approached her husband, he took one look at her and said, "Let's go. You've done too much."

  The tears were starting to come and she went in the bathroom and sobbed for a couple of minutes, got dressed, and they drove home in silence. He drew a hot bath immediately and told her to get in it. They didn't discuss it. They didn't have to. He knew how she felt and she knew he cared.

- **Remember:** Spending some time with your husband and kids is more important than a spotless house. By the way, enlist their help with housework. When you all pitch in and work together, it becomes fun and something you can all share and do together.

- Keep the lines of communication with your spouse open. He may feel resentful because you can no longer fulfill your obligations; then he feels guilty for feeling resentful. And you, the one who is in pain, probably feels guilty for not being able to take care of your responsibilities. By talking with your spouse openly, you just might be able to avoid some of the serious problems married couples encounter when one partner lives with chronic illness.

- Don't forget your children. They worry, too, when

Mommy or Daddy is hurting — don't shut them out. On the other hand, try not to let your kids see you at your worst. At certain ages, their biggest fear is losing one or both of their parents. It's frightening for them to see you in pain, depressed, and crying. You can't hide it all the time, naturally, but save your serious crying, if you can, for the privacy of your room in the comfort of your spouse's arms.

No matter how supportive your family is, sometimes it is difficult to go it alone. For some sufferers, counseling may be necessary to help the patient — and family — cope and help each other. For those who cannot afford it, the local United Way agency or your county mental health office offers a sliding scale to fit your income.

Chapter 18

Support Groups: United We Stand

With the devastation wreaked on the lives of so many TMJ sufferers, it is not surprising that The TMJ Association is constantly asked, "How do I find a support group?" or "How do I go about starting a support group?" People in pain often tend to feel isolated, partly because their doctors make them feel as though they are weird or different. Many leave jobs and withdraw from friends. They often feel no one understands. With no known cause or cure, their doctors may have told them their pain is all in their heads. Many become isolated in a world of loneliness and pain.

The Value of Support Groups

The benefits of support groups for TMJ sufferers are enormous. You will find:

- A network of people with common problems and needs can offer one another understanding, comfort, and hope.
- A safe place to vent anger and frustration and to share experiences, fears, and tears.
- Talking to others who are going through the same thing

often provides more support than family and friends, for those who have been there understand better than anyone.

- Emotional support and practical information for sufferers and their loved ones to help them feel less alone.

- Information sharing. By sharing information, sufferers and their families can deal more effectively with the multitude of problems they face every day.

- Shoulders to cry on. Talking with other TMJ patients lets you realize that you are not the only one who is suffering. You don't have to face your problems alone. Others have been there and have found ways to cope.

- A sense of warmth and caring not found in a professional environment.

- A place where you can learn to: accept your situation; keep a positive attitude; and regain control over your life.

- The positive message that you can lead a productive life in spite of your pain, or that you can at least improve your quality of life.

- You can educate yourself. People exchange information about what treatments work and don't work for them, what doctors have been helpful, and effective coping skills. With a disorder surrounded by so much controversy and doctors not agreeing on anything, sometimes the only information you can obtain is from patient to patient.

- As with any illness, if you are involved in helping others, you will think less about your own pain and problems.

- A support group gives members a sense of being represented, a sense of participating, a sense of making things happen, and a sense of lives being changed (Well Spouse Foundation) .

- **Added Bonus:** In studies of people with various illnesses, those who had attained good coping skills — often through support groups and group therapy — recovered more quickly than those who had not and actually showed higher activity of the immune system's natural "killer cells." Patients with cancer who are in therapy or belong to a support group often survive twice as long as others. Although not a cure, psychological support is a tremendous adjunct to treatment for TMJ sufferers. It can change the way you cope and therefore improve your quality of life.

The value of a support group is well expressed by one patient who wrote:

"We, who come to this support group, do so because we have lost a part of ourselves ... the loss of good health. We who come, need to be assured that it is easier to stand tall together, with people who care about us at our sides, than to stand alone. ... If you come, come knowing that you are welcomed by real people who have walked in those same new, stiff and uncomfortable shoes that you are wearing now. When you come, come with open eyes and an open heart. You will find the 'value' of your support group if you are willing to take the necessary time to look for what you need and to give to others some of what they seek" (Broock, 1991).

Another wrote: "For the first time in five, maybe eight years, I know I'm normal living in an abnormal situation."

Still another put it this way: "There is no other place in the world where people understand the life I am living."

Since the publication of the *Woman's Day* article, TMJ support groups are cropping up all over the U.S. They are being started by people who have no one who can relate to their experiences, people who want to help others who may not have any help or support and feel all alone, and people who are just sick and tired of feeling sorry for themselves and have decided to do something about it. Some are driven by a sense of outrage. Others feel they are bringing some positive action to the problem, maybe even helping to change things. And for some, forming a support group is very therapeutic. By helping others, they are helping themselves.

And TMJ patients in all phases of treatment are going to support group meetings — from those who are just beginning to those who have undergone dozens of surgeries. It is not unusual for many to burst into tears during their first visit because they have finally found other sufferers who are experiencing the same problems. Many are shocked, but relieved, to know someone else is going through a similar experience. They have gone from doctor to doctor — without getting any help. In a support group they know they can get emotional support from people who really know what it's like.

Conversation revolves around the effect TMJ has had on their lives, their relationships with families and friends, and how to deal with their anger, guilt, and depression. They talk about feelings. Day-to-day problems such as intimacy, money, children, and housework are discussed openly and freely.

People who have never met before — never even spoken on the telephone — touch, hold hands, and often cry as they share stories, ideas, and doctors' names, trying to offer hope to each other. Many leave their first meeting — after many hugs and thank-you's — knowing (perhaps for the first time) that they are not alone, that others know what they are going through. They came depressed and lonely, but they leave angry, energized, and very determined.

Instead of feeling sorry for themselves, they want to get

involved in health care reform and may even resolve to fight to get insurance coverage for their treatment. Such patients are now volunteering to work together to get more media attention, influence their senators and congressmen, and maintain a telephone support network.

Characteristics of TMJ Support Groups

- Some are fairly informal, with members determining the direction of the meetings. Others may be somewhat structured, with discussions on specific topics that may be selected by members. Or some groups try a combination of structured discussion groups and open discussion among sufferers. They may have a professional at each meeting, who can help run the meeting or in some groups, give special presentations on particular topics.

- Most groups hold regular meetings — from once a week to once a month. They meet in libraries, churches, schools, civic centers, and private homes.

- Usually, TMJ support groups are self-supporting, either through member donations or nominal dues.

- They may have more than one leader to share the load. Always, members are encouraged to become involved.

- Some groups have special meetings for the families of the sufferer. This helps them to know others are in the same situation.

- Many groups have a telephone network, a buddy system, or pen pals that allows members to have support available when it's needed the most, around the clock.

Regardless of how they are set up, support groups exist for the day-to-day support and encouragement of the members. People can reach out and touch and share with others. Sometimes a phone call from a member gives you enough hope to get through another day or night.

A successful support group has several ingredients:

"For support groups to work most effectively, members must play two roles: the helper and the "helpee." The processes of give and take, helping and being helped, caring and sharing — all these must take place for a self-help support group to help someone navigate the journey from helplessness to empowerment" (Smith, 1989).

Chapter 19

How You Can Help

1. Join The TMJ Association and become involved in our cause. Your financial support is desperately needed in order for us to continue working to bring about a change in the research and treatment direction of temporomandibular joint disorders. A lot has been accomplished, but there is still much to do. Remember: The TMJ Association is a non-profit, 501(c)(3) organization, so your donations are tax-deductible.

2. Please keep us informed about your symptoms and treatments. Tell us what this disorder has done to your quality of life and your family. We are continually learning from you and the information you share with us. We assure you we will "synthesize" this knowledge and see to it that the appropriate authorities are bombarded with it.

3. Send us a list of the names, addresses, and telephone numbers of other people you know with TMJ disorders so we can add them to our database.

4. If you know of a support group, please tell us. Be sure to include the name, address, and telephone number of the contact person. If you are a support group leader,

keep The TMJ Association up to date on your activities. If you are interested in starting a new group, let us know and we will do everything we can to help you get started.

Writing To Congress

Perhaps one of the most effective things you can do is let your Senators and Representatives know how you feel. The TMJ Association has worked with Congress in the past and we can assure you that it is the only way to get more funding for research and insurance coverage for the treatment of TMJ disorders.

Besides you, the patient, writing, it is extremely effective if family members and friends — anyone who is affected by this disorder and what it has done to their loved ones — would also write. You need to impress upon your congressmen the many ways your life has been changed because of TMJ. The list below will give you some idea of what to include.

- Do you need help to function on a daily basis, for example, to take care of your house and children, drive, go shopping, etc.?
- Are you able to hold down a job?
- Has your social life changed? If so, how?
- What effect has TMJ had on your family, for example, spouse, children, and parents?
- How has TMJ impacted on you financially? How much have you spent for treatment? Do you have insurance? If not, how are you paying for medical care? If you do have insurance, what percentage of your treatment cost is being covered?

Make your letter brief — one or two pages at the most. Send a copy to the representatives (The Honorable <u>Name</u>, U.S. House of Representatives, Washington, DC 20515) and senators (The Honorable <u>Name</u>, U.S. Senate, Washington, DC 20510) from your state and request a meeting with them to discuss this issue. After sending your letters, wait two weeks and follow up with a phone call. Be persistent! It's the only way things are going to change. Tell them to write to The TMJ Association. We will be happy to cooperate with them and provide additional information.

The following letter was written by a friend of an implant recipient. It is an excellent example of what needs to be said about the tragedy inflicted on thousands of lives as the result of a lack of TMJ research. Since the patient is involved is in a lawsuit against the implant manufacturer, the name has been changed.

"I first met Karen about five years ago. Since that time I've had the opportunity to spend quite a bit of time with her and her family. The recent years in Karen's life can be described as an endless and ongoing nightmare. I couldn't even begin to give an adequate description that would accurately reflect the full extent of Karen and her family's pain over this time period.

"Karen's deteriorating health has had a substantial impact on her ability to function on a day-to-day basis. She's had her jaw wired shut about 20 times. Her colon has been removed. She has ongoing bladder problems as well as stomach and muscle problems. I recall one occasion she was barely able to walk and eventually was forced to use a wheelchair. I've seen her suffer from ongoing sleeplessness and headaches. Because of the condition of her mouth, she has had great difficulty chewing. I've seen her smash up small pieces of hamburger in order to be able to chew them.

"Her depression and low self-esteem have been apparent. Despite her tenacious efforts to remain cheerful, hopeful, and courageous, she has fallen victim to the inevitable depression that accompanies this total physical deterioration. Her uneven smile and droopy eyes are just some of the footprints left by her many surgeries. The financial stress suffered by the family has been extreme. Karen has been unable to work. Her husband has had to take several days off work to take her to doctors' appointments and to drive her to hospitals. She often had several appointments in one day. Only some of her about 20 surgeries were covered by insurance. Some of these were performed out of state. The family has put out substantial amounts of money for surgeries and other medical care. At times they were barely able to make ends meet. At one point, her husband's wages were garnished by a medical provider.

"Karen has had an admirable attitude despite her circumstances. The jaw implant has made it difficult for her to get through each day. Although many have a lot of sympathy for Karen, few if any are capable of having empathy for her. It would be next to impossible to put oneself in her position and imagine the full extent of the emotional and physical pain she has experienced. One woman who also had a jaw implant apparently understood this pain. I'm told she committed suicide. In conclusion, I'm hopeful that all efforts are being made to halt the horrifying effects of this jaw implant for the sake of Karen and others like her."

And this next letter was written by a child who knows Karen. It's short, simple, and to the point, but it says it all:

"I am 13 years old and have known Karen for five years. Since getting the jaw implant, she has been sick a lot. It seems so unfair. Her daughter has gone through a lot because her Mom is always sick. Please don't let others' lives be ruined with them."

The TMJ Association is continuing communication with

various congressional committees that have the power to legislate insurance coverage and increase research. We need reinforcement from TMJ patients across the country to be successful. We are doing everything in our power to improve the quality of life for TMJ sufferers and ensure that we never have another implant disaster. Please help.

Chapter 20

Resources

The TMJ Association: Help and Hope

In 1986, The TMJ Association was founded in the Milwaukee area by two TMJ patients as a forum for the exchange of experiences, information, and emotional support among people with jaw joint disorders.

The group was formally incorporated in December 1989 as The TMJ Association, Ltd., a non-profit, 501(c)(3) organization with the following goals:

- To promote awareness of temporomandibular disorders among the public and professionals.

- To provide information and support for people with TMJ and their loved ones through the development of a national network of members.

- To encourage the scientific community to research the cause of TMJ and develop safe and effective treatments.

After several years of gathering information from people with TMJ disorders as well as medical professionals, we gradually began hearing from others across the country. With the growing realization that TMJ was a serious national health problem, we contacted several government agencies and professional organizations, seeking their help in our effort to address the numerous problems experienced by TMJ patients. Patient and co-founder Terrie Cowley approached the National Institute of Dental Research (NIDR), the National Institutes of Health (NIH), the Food & Drug Administration (FDA), the Congressional Women's Caucus, the American Dental Association (ADA), the American Association of Oral and Maxillofacial Surgeons (AAOMS), and congressional leaders. No one would listen to her. In June 1991, we provided public testimony to the NIH Task Force on Opportunities for Research on Women's Health concerning the status of TMJ diagnosis and treatment.

Increasingly frustrated with the lack of response from any of our efforts and convinced that congressional intervention was the only remaining alternative, in January 1992, The TMJ Association approached the U.S. Congress Subcommittee on Human Resources and Intergovernmental Relations and asked them to investigate the overall state of the art of TMJ and the danger of TMJ implants. The Committee, chaired by the late Ted Weiss (D-NY), held a congressional hearing on June 4, 1992 to review FDA and NIH policies on TMJ and jaw joint implants.

In January 1993, The TMJ Association provided testimony to a special NIDR panel urging that NIH utilize a multi-institute approach to basic research of TMJ. Recommendations made by the panel included the establishment of a new clinic to conduct research on epidemiology, etiology, diagnosis, treatment, and prevention of TMJ disorders, as well as research on biomaterials and acute and chronic pain. The panel further recommended increased collaboration among both NIDR and NIH scientists and between NIDR scientists and the extramural community.

In an effort to impress upon Congress the necessity for increased funding, in April 1993, The TMJ Association testified before the Senate Appropriations Committee, Subcommittee on Labor, Health & Human Services, and Education. Our recommendations included funding for:

- controlled scientific research
- an intensive program to educate both the public and professionals
- a national media notice of the Vitek implant recall
- a TMJ implant patient registry.

The TMJ Association's efforts resulted in report language being entered into the 1994 NIDR budget.

The TMJ Association is currently involved in a number of activities, including the following:

1. A program to develop a strong national TMJ network for the purpose of establishing a registry that will be used to explore the problems encountered by people with jaw joint disorders.

2. Plans for a national TMJ Association conference.

3. A national media campaign to increase public awareness of TMJ and the activities of The TMJ Association.

4. Maintaining communication with Congress, NIH, and the FDA to encourage research and insure that people with TMJ disorders receive safe and effective treatments.

5. Initiation of congressional contacts in an effort to help solve the insurance and financial problems which many people with TMJ face.

6. Networking with other organizations having similar objectives and concerns in order to share relevant information and collaborate on issues of mutual importance.

The TMJ Association publishes a quarterly newsletter (*The TMJ Report*) that keeps you updated on research, medical, legal, legislative, and insurance issues; provides a forum for sharing ideas and asking questions; and keeps you informed about the activities of The TMJ Association. They also maintain a list of support groups around the country. For the annual membership fee of $15, you will receive a subscription to the newsletter. Since The TMJ Association is a non-profit organization, donations are tax-deductible.

For more information about temporomandibular joint disorders, TMJ implants, and The TMJ Association, please write to:

The TMJ Association, Ltd.
6418 W. Washington Blvd.
Wauwatosa, WI 53213
(414) 259-3223

The National Chronic Pain Outreach Association

The National Chronic Pain Outreach Association (NCPOA), a non-profit organization established in 1980, is dedicated to lessening the suffering caused by chronic pain by educating pain sufferers, health care professionals, and the public about chronic pain and its management.

Experts estimate that chronic pain affects as many as one in three Americans — more than 80 million people. The most frequent types of chronic pain are back pain, arthritis, and headaches, although there are many other types. Chronic pain disables more people than cancer or heart disease and costs the U.S. economy more than $90 billion per year. Yet it has received little attention from researchers until recently and is one of the most underfunded major health problems in the United States. NCPOA operates a clearinghouse for information about chronic pain. Their services include:

- A free catalog with over 50 publications and tapes;

- A 16-page quarterly newsletter, *Lifeline*, which contains articles on pain management methods and coping skills;
- A Support Group Starter Kit to help people start local chronic pain support groups;
- A computerized Support Group Registry of chronic pain support groups in the U.S. and Canada;
- Referrals to NCPOA member health care professionals and facilities nationwide through our Referral Service.

When you join NCPOA, your membership benefits include: a subscription to their newsletter, free pamphlets, substantial member discounts on all catalog items, and access to their Support Group Registry and Referral Service. Annual dues, which are tax-deductible, are: $25 for individuals, $50 for professionals, and $100 for clinics, hospitals, and organizations.

For more information, contact:
National Chronic Pain Outreach Association (NCPOA)
7979 Old Georgetown Rd., Suite 100
Bethesda, MD 20814-2429
(301) 652-4948

Fibromyalgia Network

This organization offers a quarterly newsletter that keeps members abreast of new research findings, treatment options, and coping tips for sufferers of fibromyalgia and chronic fatigue syndrome. They also provide a list of patient support group contacts as well as physician referrals. Annual membership is $15. To find out more, contact:

Kristin Thorson
Fibromylagia Network
5700 Stockdale Hwy., Suite 100
Bakersfield, CA 93309
(805) 631-1950

The Arthritis Foundation

The mission of the Arthritis Foundation is to support research to find the cure for, and prevention of, arthritis and to improve the quality of life for those affected by arthritis.

Formed in 1948, the Arthritis Foundation is the only national, voluntary health organization that works on behalf of all people with any of the more than 100 forms of arthritis or related diseases. Volunteers in chapters nationwide help to support research, professional and community education programs, government advocacy, and fundraising activities. A wide range of helpful services exist including a bi-monthly newsletter, exercise programs, aquatics (water exercise) programs, and many, many publications. For more information, contact:

The Arthritis Foundation
1314 Spring St. NW
Atlanta, GA 30309
(404) 872-7100

Well Spouse Foundation

The too-often overlooked families of people with any type of chronic condition need help dealing with their increased responsibilities: financial, marital, and parenting difficulties; never-ending stress; and feelings of frustration, fear, anger, guilt, loneliness, worry, and helplessness. They need to know they are not alone.

In 1988, writer Maggie Strong founded the Well Spouse Foundation, a non-profit organization whose mission is "to give emotional support to, raise consciousness about, and advocate for the spouses and children of the chronically ill." They offer families much-needed information about insurance and legal issues. Their goals include changes in insurance coverage for long-term care and new programs to help families deal with chronic illness. Currently, over 70 support groups exist in the United States and new ones are being formed.

Members receive a bi-monthly newsletter, a referral to a nearby support group, help in starting a group, and telephone support. They are given understanding, a sense of belonging, and courage to cope and go on. For more information, contact:

Well Spouse Foundation
P.O. Box 801
New York, NY 10023
(212) 724-7209

Appendix

Testimony Prepared by The TMJ Association, Ltd. for the Committee on the Future of Dental Education, Institute of Medicine. Presented by the National Alliance for Oral Health, September 26, 1993.

For the past half century, temporomandibular disorder has been assigned to the dental turf. The dental schools of this country should be the intellectual driving force for basic and clinical research on TMJ disorders and the repository of all that is known about this disorder. This knowledge is transferred to all students who pass through the educational system and results in treatment modalities being carried out on patients. Unfortunately, in the area of TMJ disorders, a meta-analysis in combination with a review of the literature reveals that what is known and being taught has little scientific validity, resulting in the failure of the dental profession to provide adequate care for, and solutions to, the problems of temporomandibular joint disorder patients. How could this have happened?

Perhaps Dr. Enid Neidle, former scientific director of the American Dental Association, has the answer. She states: "Where dental schools have done an exceedingly poor job, and continue to do so, is to incorporate those things into the curriculum that will create in their graduates an inquiring mind, a respect for science, a comprehension of what research means, and a deep understanding of how fundamental to the practice of dentistry scientifically generated knowledge is." She further speculates that "our raging controversies about the ... proper diagnosis and treatment of temporomandibular disorders reflect the failure of American dental schools to provide their students with any of the resources needed to develop what can only be described as a respect for science and an ability to learn from it."

The lack of scientific integrity described by Enid Neidle has resulted in anecdotal, mythical information from which treatment modalities evolved that can be either ineffective or iatrogenically cause the disorder. This is costly, particularly to the patients in terms of diminished quality of life, and/or loss of life, family, and finances, and also to the health care system.

Because there is no known etiology of TMJ disorders, because treatment outcomes frequently do not live up to the expectations of the dentist, the patient bears the brunt of the blame. Daily we hear from patients who have been subjected to the abuses of abandonment, dumping, fraud, and deceit. But even worse is the continuous accusation of the "psychological problems." This has recently been brought to light in the ugliest sense with the TMJ implant disaster. Patients with foreign body giant cell reaction eating away the condyle and fossa to the point of skull perforations, suffering disabling systemic pathology, are being told that "nothing is wrong, its all in your head. Get out of my office and don't come back." Animals have secured more rights in this country than many TMJ patients. Dr. Michael Merson, an official of the World Health Organization, in a recent speech stated that "there is a need to understand the interplay between health and human rights." It is time this dehumanization stops.

The following are our recommendations for dental school education regarding TMJ disorders:

1. Admit to the controversy surrounding the definition, diagnosis, and treatment of TMJ disorders and the resulting damage this has caused the patients. Acknowledge the realities of the clinical, systemic, and craniofacial pathology associated with TMD, and

be honest about the limitations of the dental profession in the treatment of this disorder.

2. Solicit the appropriate basic scientists to apply their intellectual expertise and scientific protocols to TMD, and incorporate the medical professionals most qualified to treat the non-dental components of TMJ — the muscle, joint, and pain disorders — into the practice of TMJ treatment. Implied in this is the incorporation of TMJ disorders into the medical school curriculum.

We appreciate the opportunity we have had to testify on behalf of all TMJ patients. We feel strongly that our recommendations, if carried out, will be an important first step towards providing the many TMJ patients in this country with the humane care they need and deserve.

1 Enid Neidle, PhD, "On the Brink: Will Dental Education Be Ready for the Future?" Journal of Dental Education, Vol. 54, No. 9, 1990.

Testimony to the Senate Appropriations Committee, Subcommittee on Labor, Health & Human Services, and Education. Presented by Jennifer Hutchinson for The TMJ Association, April 26, 1993.

Temporomandibular disorder (TMD), commonly referred to as "TMJ," is a disorder of the jaw joint that affects one in five Americans, 80 percent of whom are women. Symptoms range from clicking and popping sounds in the joint to severe, debilitating pain and biomechanical dysfunction.

Despite the pervasiveness of this disorder, there is no consensus among professionals as to definition, cause, diagnosis, or treatment, and little research has been conducted to determine the cause of TMD or the safety and efficacy of current treatment modalities. Only two percent of the National Institute of Dental Research (NIDR) or .07 percent of the total NIH 1992 budget, was directed toward TMD research.

The absence of basic research has permitted what one researcher calls "the Great American Medical Disaster" — temporomandibular joint implants. The Proplast-Teflon implants manufactured by Vitek, Inc. were recalled in December 1990 due to their high failure rate. Some people have experienced progressive bone degeneration in as little as one or two years, resulting in chronic, excruciating pain, permanent loss of masticatory function, a broad range of immune system effects, and what the FDA says is "open communication to the brain" — meaning holes in the skull.

These implant failures have resulted in an ever-growing medical disaster. Because of the bone destruction and tissue damage caused by the implants, implant recipients will eventually need multiple revision surgeries. Many implant victims cannot afford to have their implants removed, or to pay for follow-up care, complications, and pain management. An equally distressing problem is that some of these people are seriously ill and may not even know that their implants have already failed, shattered in their heads, and are migrating throughout their bodies. The bottom line is that these people's lives have been destroyed, and little, if anything, is being done to address the numerous medical needs they will face for the rest of their lives. We offer the following recommendations:

1. That Congress direct the Department of Health and Human Services to establish a task force to determine which institutes are best able to utilize existing intellectual expertise and scientific protocols and apply them to the study of TMD. To enhance research efforts, the FDA could provide scientists with information they have obtained through their investigation of TMJ implants over the last few years. We also recommend that special funding be allocated for controlled scientific studies in the areas of epidemiology and etiology.

2. That the Department of Health and Human Services be directed to conduct a national public health media notice of the recall on Proplast-Teflon implants.

3. That NIH initiate an immediate, intensive campaign to educate both the public and professionals on the realities of this disorder and the efficacy of current treatments.

4. That a national database of TMJ implant recipients is funded. A registry will serve as an effective method for tracking these people, as well as a database from which surveys can be conducted that will allow for outcome assessment of the physical, psychological, financial, and social damage of implant recipients.

In closing, I would like to share with you the following excerpt from testimony presented by a TMJ implant victim at a congressional hearing held last summer.

"My life hasn't changed. It's gone. I feel like a big blob of pain, with big, burning-hot screws constantly twisting into my skull bone in front of my ears. This pain never goes away. It hurts to walk, it hurts to talk ... sometimes it hurts just to see. And it never stops. Every day of my life begins with thoughts of suicide. I honestly don't believe I can stand the pain much longer."

This is not an isolated case. It is almost impossible to believe that this has been allowed to happen. But it will continue to happen without research. A deplorable lack of science has left implant victims desperate and all TMD victims in "no-win" situations.

We appreciate the opportunity to speak to you today, and ask that you seriously consider our recommendations.

Testimony to the Blue Ribbon Panel on Envisioning the Future of the NIDR Intramural Research Program. Presented by Terrie Cowley for The TMJ Association, January 27, 1993.

On behalf of The TMJ Association and all people suffering from temporomandibular disorders (TMD), I thank you for providing this opportunity to speak with you.

I would like to begin by saying that I am not a scientist. I am co-founder of The TMJ Association, an organization established in 1986 in Milwaukee, Wisconsin, for the purpose of promoting awareness of this disorder among the public and professionals. We have spent the past seven years listening to the experiences of people afflicted with this disorder and the professionals involved in their treatment. Permit me to share some of what we have learned.

Conservatively speaking, each year approximately 20 percent of the population, or 52 million people, seek treatment for this disorder. Women comprise 80 to 90 percent of that number, or 43 million. In the United States, 32 billion dollars is spent on treatment of craniofacial pain annually. According to the American Dental Association (ADA), the expensive instrumentation used to aid in the diagnosis and treatment of TMD lacks well-designed scientific clinical studies upon which claims of success are based, and the clinical practice patterns show further that a wide range of TMD treatment modalities are without scientific substantiation. The lack of hard science and the financial rewards of multi-modality treatment practices have no doubt contributed to what Dr. Harold Perry sees as a greater proportion of iatrogenic problems resulting from misdiagnosis and mistreatment. The absence of science has allowed these practices to continue, and the lack of basic research in the TMD area has permitted what one researcher calls "the Great American Medical Disaster" — temporomandibular joint implants. Unfortunately, we may have only seen the tip of the iceberg in assessing the physical, psychological, and financial damage done to these people.

How has the National Institute of Dental Research (NIDR) responded to this health care need? It is obvious that, over the years, this disorder has been a low priority in interest and funding at NIDR. In 1992, only 2 percent of the budget was directed toward TMD. The majority of the funding has been to study the psychosocial ramifications of orofacial pain to the neglect of the basic science wherein most certainly should lie the pathophysiological reason for temporomandibular joint problems. It is horrifying that, in this day of sophisticated science, professionals can see the pathology of an arthritic joint, the resorption of cranial and condylar bone, giant cell reaction, evidence of proplast debris migrating through the brain, and imply that if only these people had a better attitude their pain would go away. This is dangerous medicine due to the absence of research. And the continued absence of research prohibits effective treatment solutions for all TMD patients.

It is clear that temporomandibular joint disorder is a complex, multi-faceted problem demanding the expertise of several scientific disciplines. We envision the following institutes involved with TMD research: the National Institute of Arthritis and Musculoskeletal and Skin Diseases (NIAMS), the National Institute of Allergy and Infectious Diseases (NIAID), the National Institute of Dental Research (NIDR), and the National Institute of Mental Health (NIMH). Each has expertise in some component of the TMD puzzle and we will illustrate how they can collaborate. But first, let's get down to some basic information and ways research can be applied to the temporomandibular joint.

What we have is a joint and related muscles. It would seem that if we focus research in these two areas we could gain a fundamental understanding of how the joint works and what is wrong with the muscles. Only then will we be on the way to developing treatment modalities based on science. According to other joint experts we have questioned, the following areas of study would greatly add to the meager knowledge we presently have of the jaw joint.

There is an absolute need to develop an understanding of the biomechanics of the TM joint. We need to know about the forces involved in the joint, the motion involved, and the effects of stress and strain upon the joint. We need research utilizing optimization schemes to estimate the contributions of various muscles, finite element modeling to estimate the local stresses and strains, photo-optical systems and strain gauge transducers to measure position and force. And we need to know the properties of regional TMJ tissues.

Biochemical and anatomical questions that need to be addressed include the following: What is the biochemical structure of bone and connective tissue of the TMJ? What is the metabolism of these tissues? The effect of fatigue on muscle function? What is degradation and repair of these tissues? Is there an immunological response of these tissues, for example, synovium? What happens to the blood supply and the nerve supply under mechanical disruption?

Why not develop an animal model? Why not look at normal versus abnormal joint biomechanics and biochemistry? Perhaps we should assay and culture tissue samples in normal, early and late diseased joints, as well as those with prostheses. How about comparative studies with other joints? Is it not essential that we have some comparison with other joint replacement materials and devices so we are not at risk of becoming victims once again?

NIAMS already has research protocols in place for all the areas of study just mentioned. They study all other joints and muscles in this manner. Why not the jaw joint?

The muscle disorder affiliated with TMD that affects approximately 80 percent of patients is Myofascial Pain Dysfunction (MPD) and is regional fibromyalgia. NIAMS and NIAID have jurisdiction over this disorder. Therefore, it makes sense that the institutes that have or will develop protocols for investigating fibromyalgia will essentially be researching MPD. Furthermore, the high correlation between mitral valve prolapse, joint hyperflexion, and TMD leads one to speculate that TMD is a connective tissue disorder. This falls into the realm of NIAMS. NIAID and NIAMS evaluate the immune and autoimmune processes in implant patients. The NIDR could contribute resources of the epidemiology division to finally piece together the demographics of TMD. Both NIDR and NIAMS research pain management; therefore, these two institutes could collaborate in this area. To this point, I have focused on the scientific aspect of dealing with the needs of TMD patients. Now I would like to address the devastation this disorder has wreaked on their lives. If the NIMH has no experience in helping victims of iatroepidemics, this would be a new area.

These people are living with the psychological effects of the betrayal by the FDA in allowing lethal materials to be on the market, the fraud their doctors perpetrated by selling all sorts of treatment modalities — many of which made them worse — the medical community who refuses to take seriously the medical problems of non-surgical and surgical patients and the resulting financial devastation and family disruption, and the deplorable lack of science which has left the victims desperate and in "no-win" situations. Enid Neidle, the ADA's Director of Scientific Affairs, has said that "our raging controversies ... about the proper diagnosis and treatment of temporomandibular disorders reflect the failure of American dental schools to provide their students with any of the resources needed to develop what can only be described as a respect for science and an ability to learn from it."

In light of the lack of scientific role models in the majority of dental schools, it is imperative that an attempt is made to recruit young investigators presently completing graduate and post-graduate training in medical school and bioengineering departments of the best universities. This cannot and will not happen without priority funding.

Donna Shalala, in her confirmation hearings, indicated that names put on agencies may not be appropriate for the problems they are faced with. Perhaps, in this instance, this is true. The necessity is obvious that temporomandibular disorders be appropriately placed in several institutes. We hope that NIH looks upon researching this disorder as an opportunity and a challenge. The multi-institute program we are suggesting could serve as a model for future collaboration within the Institute. More importantly, however, it will allow the best state-of-the-art science to be applied to TMD.

Public Testimony on the Current Status of TMD Diagnosis and Treatment, to the National Institutes of Health Task

Force on Opportunities for Research. Presented by Terrie Cowley for The TMJ Association, June 12-13, 1991.

It is my pleasure to present this testimony on behalf of all people afflicted with temporomandibular disorders and their loved ones who experience the frustration and anxiety of trying to make sense of a disorder that lacks consensus on definition, diagnosis, and treatment. Specifically, I represent The TMJ Association, Ltd., a non-profit organization founded in Milwaukee five years ago with the purpose of addressing the needs of TMJ patients in our community.

Temporomandibular joint syndrome (TMJ), temporomandibular disorders (TMD), and craniomandibular disorders (CMD) are some of the evolutionary terms currently used to identify this malady. For the sake of consistency, I shall use TMD in referring to it. TMD, as we see it, is a complex, multi-faceted disorder of the jaw joint, in which there is derangement of the internal mechanism and affiliated masticatory muscle pain and dysfunction. Patients may experience only the internal derangement, only the muscle pain and dysfunction, or both simultaneously. How common is TMD, who gets it and how? In a pamphlet written by the National Institute of Dental Research (NIDR), studies are cited showing a range of 10 to 77 percent of the population suffering some form of TMD. Literature yields figures of 20 to 60 million Americans having TMD. These ranges are unscientifically broad, and NIDR admits that the "discrepancies in these test results are owing, in large measure, to dental science's lack of a single definition to characterize the problem." Women account for 80 to 90 percent of TMD patients and they generally range in age from 20 to 40 years. However, professionals tell us that recently they are seeing an increasing number of teenage patients. These women represent all socio-economic levels.

The approximately 10 to 20 percent of patients who are male, have almost always experienced what is called macrotrauma —

that is, a blow to the jaw, whiplash, intubation, etc., which precipitates the joint derangement and pain. TMD's celebrity patient, Burt Reynolds, was hit in the jaw with a chair while filming a movie. This accident initiated two years of pain, vertigo, nausea, and substantial weight loss.

While in women this disorder can also be triggered by macrotrauma, the majority of female patients note gradual onset resulting from microtrauma, for example, bruxism, clenching, malocclusion, etc. NIDR states that "most TMD research has focused on identifying symptoms of the disorders, rather than the causes," and that "until more research is conducted into their causes, these conditions will remain difficult to define and often elusive to diagnose."

Despite NIDR's focus on identifying symptoms of TMD, it claims that dental scientists "have been unable to reach a consensus on what symptoms actually constitute a TMD disorder." A paper published in the mid-1980s reveals that TMD patients see on average 6.9 specialists before receiving a definitive diagnosis. The fortunate ones see only one professional. Others, like Burt Reynolds, see thirteen. The most obvious symptoms — such as joint, face, neck, back, and shoulder pain; joint clicking; popping when opening or closing the mouth — lend themselves to a fairly direct diagnosis. However, remote symptoms, including visual disturbances, ataxia, hearing loss, and vertigo, can lead a patient from one doctor to another to undergo expensive batteries of tests that yield negative results and leave the patient increasingly frightened and frustrated.

The lack of definition and diagnostic criteria has encouraged both the underdiagnosis as well as the overdiagnosis of TMD. One adult patient suffered excruciating head pain when she was 10 years old. She was sent from one mental institution to another for a period of six years until an internal derangement of the jaw was diagnosed. Another woman suffered debilitating headaches for six years. She mentioned this to her dentist, who diagnosed a TMD problem. After two years of orthodontics and another two years of combined orthodontic and splint therapies, she went to Mayo Clinic, where she learned that her headaches were vascular in origin, caused by estrogen replacement therapy.

The American Dental Association (ADA) states that 80 percent of patients get better with or without treatment. In fact, a recent study shows that more patients fare better on professional advice and home treatment, such as hot and cold packs, soft diet, and aspirin, than those who receive more extensive and costly treatment, such as splint, pharmacological, and physical therapies, as well as psychological counseling. Are patients getting better because of treatment or in spite of treatment? We don't know. Are patients being introduced to life-long chronic pain because of treatment? We can only guess.

The FDA reports that all diagnostic and treatment instrumentation for TMD lacks scientific validity. The ADA says that the claimed benefits of diagnostic instrumentation and treatment modalities are unproven. NIDR states that there is no solid scientific understanding of the causes of TMD and, with no standardized curriculum to educate dentists on the subject, diagnosis and treatment of TMD has become an area of controversy. The literature is filled with statements such as the following: "Rarely in the history of dentistry have so many labored so long only to end with such extreme disagreement."[1] "Few afflictions have spawned so much vocal controversy within the scientific community, where available treatments — some grounded in science, others of questionable value — are more numerous than symptoms."[2] This is the state of the art of TMD.

An inherent dilemma of TMD is that it crosses the boundaries of two disciplines — dentistry and medicine. Greater interaction between the two professions is necessary in both the treatment and research of TMD if progress is to be made. Cooperation and joint effort could hasten solutions to the many questions surrounding TMD. In the meantime, what of the women of this country who do not get better, with or without treatment? The women who develop a chronic or remittent course of craniomandibular dysfunction? These women are making a valiant attempt to lead functional lives in the home and workplace while living in a nightmare of pain, uncertainty, and misunderstanding. At this time they face years of their lives spent in doctors' and dentists' offices and pain clinics. Because they are in pain and are desperate, they often fall prey to the latest hit-or-miss treatments that sound like voodoo medicine.

They will spend thousands of dollars on scientifically unproven treatment modalities and, months and years later, end up poorer, no better, and perhaps worse. They may undergo surgical procedures and later learn that an implant provoked not only condyle and skull disintegration but also giant cell neoplasia, opening the door to multiple surgeries. Their insurance companies will reject the claims because they say there are no standards for diagnosis or treatment. Their professional health-care providers will look at them and say, "We did everything we could. We don't know why you aren't getting better." I think our women deserve better.

I truly hope this brief overview will encourage NIH to make a commitment to the many TMD sufferers of this country. We request:

1. An intensive program to educate both patients and professional providers as to the realities of this disorder and current treatment efficacy.

2. Focused research on the following:

    a. Epidemiology of non-patient population base as well as patient population.

    b. Etiology — from the molecular, biomechanical, neuroendocrine as well as physiological and clinical perspectives.

3. Development of treatment programs based on solid scientific research.

Sources

[1] Greene, C.S. "Myofascial Pain-Dysfunction Syndrome: The Evolution of Concepts," Chapter 13, In *The Temporomandibular Joint.* Edited by B.G. Sarnat, and D.M. Laskin. Charles C. Thomas, Springfield, IL, 1980

[2] "The Traumas of TM," *ADA News*, Sept. 5, 1988, p. 1.

Testimony Presented Before the Subcommittee on Human Resources & Intergovernmental Relations, Committee on Government Operations, U.S. House of Representatives, 102nd Congress, 2nd Session, June 4, 1992.

Theresa Cowley, Wauwatosa, Wisconsin

Good morning. I am Terrie Cowley, co-founder of The TMJ Association, Ltd., and I am here to testify about my experiences with silicone jaw joint implants and the experiences of other people with other types of jaw joint implants.

Nearly 15 years ago, I was told by my physicians that the frequent headaches that I was experiencing were due to my jaw joints. It was found that the discs which normally cushion the movement of the jaw joint into my skull were perforated and that degenerative arthritis had developed in both joints. After five years of continuing discomfort, I underwent a surgical procedure in 1982 in which both of the discs were removed and replaced with Dow Corning silicone jaw joint implants.

From the day of surgery, my condition worsened. For nearly three years, I experienced excruciating headaches, neck and back pain, and extreme fatigue. My vision and hearing were distorted. I developed problems of balance and equilibrium. I encountered memory lapses and a reduction of my ability to articulate. I could no longer function well enough to maintain a full-time job and lived in a state of terror, not knowing how long I could live in a continually worsening physical state. I was passed from one professional to another, none of whom could offer any help.

In 1986, four years after my surgery, I met another jaw joint patient and we formed The TMJ Association, Ltd. It has been our goal to obtain as much information as possible about this disorder from patients and professionals. We also want to provide a way so other patients could meet and support each other. Finally, we want to promote awareness of this disorder in the community.

In the past six years I have been from one end of the country to the other, talking with patients and professionals to learn about the causes and treatments and life experiences of people suffering from this disorder. I learned that jaw joint disorders are quite common and that I was one of nearly 12 to 28 percent of the population (30 to 50 million people) that annually seeks treatment for this disorder. Nearly 90 percent of these are female and, although it has not been yet determined how many have undergone surgery and / or disc replacement, it is clear that they number in the hundreds of thousands.

Yet, despite the pervasiveness of this disorder, it remains ill defined by the dental and medical professions and there are raging controversies over diagnosis and treatment.

In the last few years I have talked to many patients with jaw joint disorders. I constantly hear what scientists call anecdotes and what I call horror stories. I talk daily to patients with stories similar to those of patients you will hear testify today. They tell of broken marriages because their spouses cannot cope with the unending pain and disability.

They tell of the financial burden placed on them and their family members to the point of bankruptcy. In a recent conversation with a lawyer, I was told that 57 of her 60 temporomandibular joint implant clients were either bankrupt or so financially compromised that they were close to bankruptcy. They tell of constant pain so severe that every day is a battle against suicide.

They tell of the inability of even their physicians to relate to their pain, such as the patient who was told to "go home, have a few drinks, make love, and forget you have pain." And they tell me that they live in terror because their symptoms indicate that the implant material has worked its way into the brain and they do not have the money to have it removed. These are the people who have begged me to find a way to tell other victims about this disaster "before they get like I am."

I found that people who have this disorder become isolated. They become isolated from their children, because the children have learned to go to others for their basic needs. They become isolated in the marital sense from their husbands, for intimacy many times takes second place to pain and even the simple act of hugging is painful. They become isolated from society, never being able to plan on such simple things like going to a movie or taking a trip because they never know if they will be physically well enough. They become isolated from the professional providers. A pain management specialist once told me that the TMJ patients are the most tragic of all. When I asked why, he said that "everybody treats them, they rarely get better, and there is no one professional who assumes responsibility for the treatment."

Because there is no known etiology for jaw joint disorders, it is not uncommon to identify this disorder as psychogenic in origin and suggest the sufferer may be responsible for the cause and/or maintenance of his or her pain. In fact, at a recent meeting, I heard a speaker state that all his patients get psychological evaluations, but of course we call it pain management.

The stigma is apparent. Last year at an NIH workshop on Women's Research in cardiovascular disease that I attended with my husband, breakfast conversation focused on jaw joint disorders. The scientists easily discussed what they thought were reasons for the disorder, while the only woman at the table remained silent. Later, she took me aside and told me she had the disorder but she would never let her peers know because they would think she was crazy. And, I also hear from the minority with this disorder — the men. The men who are afflicted are suffering in silence. They hesitate to attend a meeting or to ask for help.

Although my own symptoms have gradually lessened, I am left with the same dilemma that many other patients now face. My implants have fractured and fragmented and I have pieces of silicone in my joints which are causing constant inflammatory responses with facial swelling and pain. The other symptoms wax and wane. So why don't I simply have the implants removed? Daily I weigh the benefits and risks of having the implants taken out: an outcome surgical outcome, with no viable options for an implant replacement, and on the other hand knowing that the implants continue to break and cause my jaw bones to degenerate.

I have gone to the National Institute of Dental Research, the NIH Office of Research on Women's Health, the FDA, the Agency for Health Care Policy and Research, the Congressional Women's Caucus, the American Dental Association, the American Association of Oral and Maxillofacial Surgeons, and other professional and congressional leaders, seeking their attention to this problem. I am most grateful that this congressional hearing, Mr. Chairman, represents a serious effort to examine the disastrous state of the art of diagnosis and treatment of this disorder and the lack of serious efforts to deal with it.

What can be done? It is my hope that recognition of these problems will lead to:

First, a public health notice of recall on Proplast/Teflon (Vitek, Houston, TX) implants should be widely publicized in both print and on TV. A national center should be established to develop a database based on a registry of patients who have received any type of alloplastic TMJ implant. The FDA, the Arthritis Institute, and the National Institute of Dental Research, must collaborate to conduct controlled, coordinated studies of patients who have received Proplast/Teflon, Silastic implants, or other TMJ implants, to determine the extent of damage to the jaw and skull and systemic pathology. Collaborative efforts between federal agencies and the device and materials industry is necessary to address the needs of the large number of TMJ implant patients.

Second, a serious effort to educate patients and professional providers as to the realities of this disorder and current treatments, is needed.

Third, federally funded research should be initiated to better characterize the nature and causes of this disorder, as well as the development of methods of treatment based on solid scientific research.

Amy Marks, New Orleans, Louisiana

My name is Amy Marks. The pain is so bad it is hard for me to know where to begin. Tuesday, I was released from the hospital, where I was being treated for pain control. I feel useless, like I'm just taking up space.

I developed TMJ problems in 1979 after an automobile accident. I have had 19 surgeries to date, and still I have to fill my body up with pain pills, anti-inflammatories, and muscle relaxers just to get through the day — which is still no more than lying in bed in agony. The surgeries I had in 1983, 1984, and 1986 changed my life forever. The hour or hour and a half it took to place the Proplast Teflon in my head have proven to be irreversible. My life has come to a halt. The implants shattered, and today, tiny particles of Teflon are floating around in my head causing severe, constant pain.

Once the implants failed, everything after that was doomed.

The Teflon made my jaw joint fail, and the doctors kept trying to rebuild it with two of my ribs and a collar bone. It took a lot of energy, strength, and courage to face each surgery. I thought each would be my last, and would give me back my life, so I kept agreeing to them. This is the point when suicide first entered my mind.

Every graft dissolved — a reaction which I have learned is common among Proplast survivors. A Christensen joint, made by TMJ Implants, failed so badly that the end of it stuck out of the side of my head. Before receiving my TechMedica joints, I lived without a jaw at all, which was extremely painful and disfiguring. I have scars and aching bones all over my body where bone and skin grafts were taken, as reminders of all these failures.

If Vitek, Methodist Hospital, Dupont, LSU Medical School, Dr. John Kent, or the FDA had come out a few years ago and admitted these problems, I could have avoided several failed surgeries.

Jaw surgery is major surgery, and it is extremely difficult and painful. Recovery takes weeks, followed by very painful physical therapy. I have been so weak and depressed, and at 5-8" have gotten down to 69 pounds, that I had to crawl to get to the bathroom because I was too weak to walk.

At one point, the pain and medication affected my body so much that my husband and I were told that I had AIDS. Of course, AIDS is not an issue. These symptoms were caused by the pain, the jaw problems, and the medical treatment.

Because this is an unseen illness, I have been shamed and degraded by doctors and nurses who didn't believe me. They said I was just a drug addict, or told me what I needed was a psychiatrist because the pain was in my head. After one surgery, my pain pump was mistakenly set at one-tenth of the medication I was prescribed. The nurses kept telling me to stop complaining, that I had developed a tolerance to the medication and they were giving me all they could.

I don't know what's worse — the pain itself, or the emotional pain of being trapped in a body that can't function. It takes a lot of energy to manage the pain, and it leaves me feeling very vulnerable with no resources for me to fall back on. I have easily bought into the accusations and wondered, What is wrong with me? Why can't I just snap out of it? Why am I letting pain control my life — as if I have a choice in it. I start discounting myself.

Having children is a decision that has been taken away from me. With the amount of medication I am on I couldn't safely carry a child. I am beyond anger. I'm devastated, all because of a small piece of plastic.

I have tried many other treatments besides surgery, including acupuncture, biofeedback, cortisone shots, splint therapy, and physical therapy. In one series of shots, local anesthetics were injected into 10 or 12 points of my head every week. I've been hospitalized for up to three weeks at a time for pain control. I've been given life-threatening levels of narcotics until I could barely talk, but there was still pain.

Today, I have TechMedica metal jaw joints on both sides of my head. Although the joints seem fine, the inflammation and scarring in the surrounding tissue severely limit my mouth opening and cause constant, agonizing pain. I can eat only must, and even that increases my pain so much that I'm often confined to bed after a meal.

As a result of the surgeries, my face is partially paralyzed. It is also somewhat deformed because some of my jaw muscles are permanently severed. But the worst part is the swelling on both sides of my face. It is the constant, painful inflammation of a jaw that does not heal.

My life hasn't changed. It's gone. I feel like a big blob of pain, with big, burning-hot screws constantly twisting into my skull bone in front of my ears. This pain never goes away. Sometimes I also get sudden, sharp, stabbing pain that causes me to drop whatever is in my hands, shut my eyes, and hold on to something to keep from falling. The pain and medication have reduced my blood pressure so much that I pass out and fall down. It hurts so much I can't drive, read, or do anything that requires thought or concentration for more than a few minutes. It hurts to walk, it hurts to talk for too long a time. Sometimes it hurts just to see. And it never stops.

I didn't ask for this. I could be anyone. Your wife, or your daughter. Before I entered this hell on earth, I was a dynamic, very productive person. I was a fashion model. I kept the books for several showrooms in the World Trade Center in Dallas. I ran a successful greenhouse and plant store. I managed a trendy upscale restaurant in Dallas, where I worked 20-hour days. I was an artist, a jewelry designer, and an interior decorator.

Now, I can't concentrate enough to read a book, balance a checkbook, or write more than a few sentences. I can only eat mush, and even that is agony. I depend on others for my most basic needs. Suicidal thoughts are not from an occasional depression. That's how I start every day. I pray for the emotional strength to get out of bed, and not be so angry.

In addition, my life is lonely. I used to have so many friends, but now I am trapped in my bedroom. I miss seeing and talking to other people. I miss giving my husband passionate kisses. I miss the freedom of getting out of bed whenever I want to, the freedom of driving a car, the freedom of going wherever I want to, of going anywhere alone. Basically, I miss the freedom that healthy people take for granted. Everything I do, I must plan and prepare so the medicine is working at just the right time. And then it always wears off before I'm ready. Watching a movie is even difficult because it's hard for me to concentrate.

I am trying to find the money and a doctor to have a pain pump implanted in my stomach. It will constantly infuse morphine into my spine. One anesthesiologist thinks this temporary measure will reduce the pain enough for me to leave my house on my own. Otherwise, I honestly don't believe I can stand the pain much longer.

Unfortunately, no doctor wants the responsibility of treating me. They all seem scared of my complex case and unwilling to accept what little insurance I have left.

The financial burden has been almost as devastating as the pain. I have creditors calling daily to collect on bills the insurance doesn't cover. I am 36 years old, and I've been unable to work for years. My parents are using up their retirement money. My family loves me and the money could be tolerated if we didn't feel we were throwing it into a black hole of empty lies and broken promises.

Even with these problems, I checked out of the hospital against my doctor's wishes and paid my own way here today. I feel like the years since 1983 have left me feeling useless, completely unproductive and trapped in my body of pain. This testimony gives my life purpose. Even though I've only been given five minutes to speak, I feel it is the most important five minutes of my life. I came because those of us who suffer TMJ and Proplast Teflon poisoning need help and deserve answers.

- We want to know why these implants were allowed on the market.
- Why weren't they properly tested?
- Why were they just taken off the market a year ago, when there was so much evidence against them earlier?
- Why aren't the designers, manufacturers, and marketers of these implants, and those in government who approved them, being held accountable for destroying my life and thousands of other lives?
- Why is it that neither the FDA nor the National Institutes of Health have funded research into TMJ and implants?
- Why aren't there funds available to help me and thousands like me who are suffering?

But mostly, my hope and my final prayer is that you will make the money available for the research to neutralize the effects on my body from Proplast.

Doctors, hospitals, the federal government, the FDA, and the NIH all have failed me and thousands of others who suffer because of a little piece of plastic. I hope this testimony isn't in vain. What's my purpose in living if I can't do anything to make my life worthwhile? This cannot wait. We must have action — I must have hope — NOW.

Paula Beaulieu, Tualatin, Oregon

Mr. Chairman and members of the subcommittee. My name is Paula Beaulieu and I live in Tualatin, Oregon. I would like to thank you for this opportunity to relate to you the tragedy of my life in regards to Vitek Proplast/Teflon and Dow Corning Silastic TMJ implants.

I have experienced chronic and debilitating pain since 1985, when my Proplast implant was placed. Chronic pain dictates my life, and affects every aspect of my daily living. I have pain with every movement of my jaw.

I have undergone 17 TMJ surgeries since 1981; 15 of those surgeries are directly related to the placement of Vitek's Proplast/Teflon implant in 1985, and Dow Corning's Silastic implant in 1988. Multiple surgeries have changed me from a happy, fun-loving person, to someone who is consumed with catastrophic health problems.

As a result of retained Teflon fragments, which could not be completely removed surgically, my body has reacted by destroying the top of my jaw bone and some of my skull. Over the years, I developed a receded chin and a gross open bite, and was unable to close my mouth. I lost the ability to chew solid food and my speech became severely impaired.

Besides looking like a freak, I became totally dysfunctional. Doctors have utilized muscles from my skull and cartilage from my ears, trying to restore the function of my jaw. I have sustained nerve injury to my face, as a result of multiple surgeries.

Every surgery was a failure, and my pain continued. Sometimes my pain would be so bad, that I couldn't get up, except to vomit. I have always been an active person and enjoyed working in the medical and dental field. Because of my problems with these implants, I have lost the ability to obtain or maintain full-time employment.

In August 1990, a radical form of surgery was proposed to me. The oral surgeon wanted to cut two ribs out of my chest and graft them into my jaw. He told me that my jaw bone was continuing to erode, due to the retained materials from the previous implants. I shuddered at the thought of having my ribs cut out of my chest, and I couldn't bring myself to consent to this radical procedure.

In desperation, I went to the local university medical library and began researching prosthetic joints, where I found an article about a company named "TMJ Implants," founded by Dr. Bob Christensen. "TMJ Implants" manufactures a prosthetic joint replacement for the jaw.

After consulting with Dr. James Curry in Colorado, I decided to have the TMJ replacement surgery. In December 1990, I underwent eight hours of intense reconstructive surgery to replace my TMJ. I now have 24 screws and 4 metal plates in my skull.

The surgery was partially successful, in that it restored my face by giving me back my chin and allowing me to close my mouth. I still continue to have chronic and sometimes debilitating pain, but because I look fairly normal it makes my burden easier to bear.

As I speak to you today, I am in need of additional surgery due to bone growth in and around my prosthetic joints. I have to pry my mouth open with my fingers many times throughout the day. I literally rip and tear bony tissue as I manipulate my jaw, and it is very painful.

My TMJ prosthetic joints are functioning properly. In my opinion, my continuing problems are a direct result of the original injuries caused by the Vitek Proplast/Teflon implant.

My family has had to sacrifice their lives for mine, both physically and financially, and without their support and encouragement, I may well have ended my life.

Since the placement of the Vitek implant in 1985, my medical expenses have exceeded $172,000 and my out-of-pocket expenses have exceeded $40,000. My medical expenses will continue for the balance of my life, and I expect my future medical expenses will be over one million dollars.

There are thousands of who have had the Vitek Proplast/Teflon and/or Dow Corning Silastic implants. We are facing a lifetime of surgery, medical expenses, and pain. I am scared, but I will prevail.

References

American Academy of Pediatric Dentistry, University of Texas Health Science Center, San Antonio Dental School. "Treatment of Temporomandibular Disorders in Children: Summary Statements and Recommendations." *Journal of the American Dental Association*, Vol. 120, March 1990.

American Dental Association. "Revised Draft Status Report on Devices for the Diagnosis and Treatment of Temporomandibular Disorders," Jan. 15, 1989.

Antczak, Alexia. In Sandra Blakeslee's "Routine Removal of Wisdom Teeth Wastes Millions, Report Contends," *New York Times*, June 26, 1991.

Berry, James. "Questionable Care: What Can Be Done About Dental Quackery?" *Journal of the American Dental Association* 115: 679-685, Nov. 1987.

Bosanquet, A.G.; J. Ishimaru; A.N. Goss. "The Effect of Silastic Replacement Following Discetomy in Sheep TMJ." *Journal of Oral and Maxillofacial Surgery*, Vol. 49, 1991.

Broock, Sabra. "New Kid on the Block." *Joint Adventure*. San Diego County Chapter, Arthritis Foundation, 1991.

Carerra, G.F., MD. "Diagnostic Imaging of the Temporomandibular Joint," *The TMJ Report*, Vol. 2, No. 2, May 1992.

Dodes, John, DDS. Telephone Interview, Oct. 30, 1991.

Dodes, John, DDS; Stephen Barrett, MD, Editor. "Dubious Dental Care," Special Report, American Council on Science and Health, April 1991.

Dolwick, M.F.; T.B. Audermorte. "Silicone Induced Foreign Body Reaction and Lymphadenopathy After TMJ Arthroplasty." *Oral Surgery, Oral Medicine, and Oral Pathology*, Vol. 59, 1985.

Dutson, Henry, DDS. Personal Interview, April 1988.

Dutson, Henry, DDS. Telephone Interview, June 1991.

Dutson, Henry, DDS. "TMJ and the Insurance Dilemma," *The TMJ Report*, Vol. 1, No. 7, Oct. 1991.

Fontenot, Mark, DDS, M.Eng. Testimony Before the Human Resources and Intergovernmental Relations Subcommittee, Committee on Government Operations, U.S. House of Representatives, June 4, 1992.

Food & Drug Administration. "TMJ Implants: A Consumer Information Update," Aug. 1993.

Fricton, James, DDS. "Recent Advances in Temporomandibular Disorders and Orofacial Pain, *Journal of the American Dental Association*, Vol. 122, Oct. 1991.

The Functional Orthodontist, Vol. 1, No. 4, Nov./Dec. 1984.

Gendleman, Jill. "Sex and Chronic Pain: The Healing Touch." *Lifeline*, National Chronic Pain Outreach Association, Feb. 1989.

Gordon, M; P.G. Bullough. "Synovial and Osseous Inflammation in Failed Silicone Rubber Prostheses." *Journal of Bone and Joint Surgery*, Vol. 64, 1982.

Lader, E.; L. Vander. "Insurance Coverage for the Treatment of Craniomandibular Disorders." *Dental Clinics of North America*, Vol. 31, 1987.

Lappe, Mark, PhD. Testimony Before the Human Resources and Intergovernmental Relations Subcommittee, Committee on Government Operations, U.S. House of Representatives, June 4, 1992.

Laskin, Daniel, DDS. "Assuming Our Responsibilities." *Journal of Oral and Maxillofacial Surgery*, Vol. 51, 1993.

Loe, Harald, DDS. Keynote Address, Scientific Congress on Orofacial Pain and Temporomandibular Disorders. Scottsdale, AZ, Feb. 12, 1993.

Long, James, MD. *The Essential Guide to Prescription Drugs 1993*. New York: HarperCollins, 1993.

Marbach, Joseph, DDS. "Clicks, Cracks, Crackles and Pops: The Great TMJ Pandemic." *Executive Health Report,* Vol. 22, No. 12, Sept. 1986.

Marbach, Joseph, DDS. "Losing Face: Sources of Stigma as Perceived by Chronic Facial Pain Patients." *Journal of Behavioral Medicine,* Vol. 13, No. 6, 1990.

Marbach, Joseph, DDS. Telephone Interview, July 7, 1993.

Marbach, Joseph, DDS. "The 'Temporomandibular Pain Dysfunction Syndrome' Personality: Fact of Fiction?" *Journal of Oral Rehabilitation,* Vol. 19, 1992.

Marbach, Joseph, DDS. Testimony Before the Human Resources and Intergovernmental Relations Subcommittee, Committee on Government Operations, U.S. House of Representatives, June 4, 1992.

Marbach, Joseph, DDS. "The Validity of Tooth Grinding Measures: Etiology of Pain Dysfunction Syndrome Revisited." *Journal of the American Dental Association,* Vol. 120, March 1990.

McCarty, William, DMD. Personal Interview, April 1988.

McNeill, Charles, DDS, et al. "Temporomandibular Disorders: Diagnosis, Management, Education, and Research." *Journal of the American Dental Association,* Vol. 120, March 1990.

National Institute of Dental Research. "Temporomandibular Disorders." NIH Publication No. 94-3487.

Neidle, Enid, PhD. "On the Brink: Will Dental Education Be Ready for the Future?" *Journal of Dental Education,* Vol. 54, No. 9, 1990.

Parker, Michael, DMD. "A Dynamic Model of Etiology in Temporomandibular Disorders." *Journal of the American Dental Association,* Vol. 120, March 1990.

Perry, Harold, DDS. "Above All Else, Do No Harm." *Journal of Craniomandibular Disorders: Facial and Oral Pain* 5(2): 8, 1991.

Remba, Zev. "Fraud in Dentistry." *AGD Impact*, Vol. 15, No. 7, Aug.-Sept. 1987.

Rugh, John, PhD; William Solberg, DDS. "Oral Health Status in the United States: Temporomandibular Disorders," *Journal of Dental Education*, Vol. 49, No. 6, 1985.

Ryan, Doran, DDS. "Temporomandibular Disorders." *Current Opinion in Rheumatology*, Vol. 5, 1993.

Smith, Jinx. "Caring, Sharing, and Coping: Today's Support Groups Really Work!" *Lifeline*, National Chronic Pain Outreach Association, Aug. 1989.

Tilghman, Donald, DDS. Personal Correspondence, Feb. 1994.

Weinberg, Lawrence, DDS; Jack Chastain, DMD. "New TMJ Clinical Data and the Implication of Diagnosis and Treatment." *Journal of the American Dental Association*, Vol. 120, March 1990.

Weiss, Ted, Chairman. Human Resources & Intergovernmental Relations Subcommittee, Committee on Government Operations, U.S. House of Representatives, June 4, 1992.

Well Spouse Foundation, brochure, New York, NY.

Wolford, Larry, DDS. Testimony Before the Human Resources & Intergovernmental Relations Subcommittee, Committee on Government Operations, U.S. House of Representatives, June 4, 1992.

Yates, John, MD; Elizabeth Wallace. *The Complete Book of Self-Hypnosis*. New York: Ballantine, 1984.

Zaejian, Julie. "Insurance Coverage Spotty for TMJ Care, Part III." *Daily Freeman*, Kingston, NY, July 30, 1991.

Index

Order another copy of *The Truth About TMJ*

Call our Toll-free number:

800-303-2244

VISA and Master Card accepted

TO ORDER BY MAIL:

Send check or money order for **$14.95 + $1.05 shipping ($16.00 Total) to:**

Reinhardt & Still Publishers
Box 3232
Winchester, VA 22604

Please send me _____ copies of *The Truth About TMJ : How to Help Yourself.*   Enclosed is $ _____

Name: _____

Address: _____

City: _____ State: _____ Zip: _____